Neuro-Linguistic Programming

Read People And Think Positively And Successfully Using NLP to Kill Negativity, Procrastination, Fear And Phobias (Body Language, Positive Psychology, Productivity)

Adam Hunter

Table Of Contents

Table Of Contents 3

Introduction 1

Chapter One: What is NLP? 5

   Inception 5

   Expansion of the Development Team 6

   Books, Workshops, and More 8

   The Commercialization of NLP 9

   The Current State of NLP 9

   Uses of NLP 10

      Personal Life 10

      Professional Life 10

      Social Life 11

Chapter Two: Identify & Evaluate 13

   Worry About the Future 13

   Worry About the Present 14

   Shame in Your Past 15

Chapter Three: The Power of the Subconscious Mind 17

Chapter Four: NLP Training 23

   Neuro 23

   Linguistic 24

   Programming 24

   Techniques 25

      Association – Music 25

      The Trigger 26

Daily Affirmations..26
Kill the Voices..27
The Whiteout...27
Grounding 28
Take Words at Face Value....................................29
Experimentation 30
Anchoring..30
Pacing 32
The Pizza-Walk 32
Mirroring...33
The Swish 34

Chapter Five: NLP – Higher Level of Thinking 36

Using NLP for Yourself 36

The Map isn't the Territory...................................37
There is No Failure...37
Communication and its Response 38
You Cannot Fail to Communicate........................38
Dissociate Yourself..39
Reframe 39
Anchor Yourself...40
Build Rapport..40
Limiting Beliefs 40

Use NLP on Others.. 40

The Antipodean Lilt 41
Embedded Commands..41
Restricting the Choice...42
"I can, but I'd Rather Not" 43
Know When to Use "and" and "but" 44
Find out What People really Want........................45

Chapter Six: Explaining VAK................................ 47

Understanding Nonverbal Cues 48

Facial Expressions..48
Eye Contact 49
Mouth 49
Posture 49
Touch...49

Tone 50

Understanding Context 50

The Conversation 51
The Surrounding Area during the Conversation: 51
Recent Experiences: 51
Smile 52
Eye Contact 52
Jittery Movements 52
Posture 53
Placement of Legs 53
Placement of Hands 53

Facial Expressions 54

Eyes 54

Gazing 54
Blinking 55
Size of the Pupil 55

Mouth 55

Pursed Lips 56
Biting of the Lip 56
Covering of the Mouth 56
Gestures 56

Arms and Legs 57

Postures 57

Open Posture 57
Closed Posture 58

Personal Space 58

Intimate Distance 58
Personal Distance 58
Social Distance 58

Chapter Seven: NLP and Anchoring 60

Steps to Create an Anchor 67

Pick a Memory 67
Association 67
The Feeling 67

Release..68
Test..68
Repeat..68

Chapter Eight: NLP for Procrastination and Negative Beliefs Specifically..69

NLP for Procrastination..69

NLP to Overcome Negative Beliefs 70

Dealing with Life...74

Making a Conscious Decision.................................76

Separate Your Thoughts 76

Who is Thinking those Thoughts? 76

Chapter Nine: NLP for Fear and Phobias.................78

Overcome Fear and Hesitation 78

Overcome Phobias 83
Avoid 83
Desensitization...83
Flooding 84

Chapter Ten: Other Ways to Support Positive Thinking 86

Get Sufficient Sleep...86

Healthy Eating Habits 86

Drink Plenty of Water 87

Don't Forget to Treat Yourself 88

Friends Matter..88

Smile Often 89

Enjoy Your Hobbies 89

Stay Away from Negative People 90

Don't Forget the Important Things in Life 90

Chapter Eleven: Maintaining Positivity.....................*92*

Overcome Obstacles.. 92

Focus on the Result 92
Define What You Want to Accomplish 92
Make a Note of the Reasons...92
If You Don't Do It 93
Setting Mini Goals 93
Scheduling 93
Marking Your Progress...93

Staying Consistent 94

Make a to-Do List 94
Create a Reward System...94
Breaking Up Your Workday 94
Don't Indulge in Any Activities that will Waste Your Time..................94
Tackle the Tough Tasks First 95
Discuss Your Goals with Someone 95

Kill Procrastination *95*

Figure Out the Reason..95
Getting Rid of the Obstacle 96
Just Get Started 96
Break it Down 96
The Right Environment...97
Rejoice in the Small Victories 97
Be Realistic 97
Self-Talk...98
Don't Try to be a Perfectionist 98

Chapter Twelve: Homework 99

One Problem per Day.. 99

Internalizing Intellectual Standards 100

Maintain an Intellectual Journal 100

Reshaping Your Character 101

Dealing with Your Egocentrism 101

Redefining the Way in which You See Things.................102

Get in Touch with Your Emotions 102

Analyzing the Influence of a Group on Your Life...........103
    One Door Shuts and the Other Opens 103
    The Gift of Time 103
    Counting Kindness 104
    The Funny Things 104
    Letter of Gratitude 104
    The Good Things 104
    Making Use of Your Signature Strengths 104

Conclusion.. 105

Resources 109

Introduction

I thank you for choosing this book, Neuro-Linguistic Programming: Become the Person You Want to be Using NLP by Training your Brain to Think Positively to Create a Successful Life, and I hope you have a good time reading it.

In this age of cutthroat competition, it becomes all the more important that people utilize their mental capacity optimally to achieve success. Not doing so might leave you behind while your competitors surge forward. All human beings have the potential to multitask and can complete arduous tasks in no time. Not everyone is capable of doing this, and only those who realize their true mental potential, by training their mind to work at its optimal level, will be able to attain the success they dream of.

There will always be those who excel in their chosen field, and then there will be those who look up to them in envy. If everybody fell into the former category, then there would be no competition in this world; however, the main goal for a lot of us is to come out on top and leave the competition behind. So, what is it that differentiates the winners, and what do others lack? Well, the answer to this question lies in a simple concept: NLP.

Certain skills like self-confidence, good communication skills, and leadership abilities are important to be successful in all aspects of your life—personal as well as professional. For a lot of people, it is a necessity, and the lack of these qualities can make them feel inferior. Even if you possess all these skills, we can all use a good boost of self-confidence once in a while, but there is a small problem. The boost mentioned here is not available in the form of a tablet or a pill that you can purchase at your local drugstore. The only way to acquire it is by stepping out of your shell and summoning these qualities from within yourself. This is where NLP steps in.

NLP refers to neuro-linguistic programming, and it is a simple concept that allows a person to control their mind, and those of others, while influencing thoughts and behaviors to gain more out of life.

Well, why do you want to learn about NLP? Have you ever noticed that you are overcome with a wide range of negative emotions? Do you feel like your fears or your phobias control your life? Do you wonder where your negative emotions are sprouting from? Are you tired of looking at things through a vision that's tinted with negativity? Are you tired of all this, and do you want to change? If your answer is yes to all these questions or any one of them, then NLP can help you.

The world that we live in is overwrought with negative emotions. Negative emotions are those internal feelings that make us feel bad about ourselves and those around us. Negative emotions can be quite a hindrance when you want to achieve success in life. Well, here is a small secret about negative emotions: you can control them. Yes, you can control all that you feel, and you don't have to be a victim of your emotions. There are certain negative emotions that are generated in response to someone else. For instance, greed, envy, jealousy, or even hatred are often generated as a response to someone else's behavior. Do you ever find yourself feeling jealous of your colleague who seems to be doing well for himself even if you both do the same work? Negative emotions can also be a result of your internal feelings. For instance, your fears, doubt, lack of confidence, and such can also prevent you from achieving the success you want. Fears and phobias can prevent you from taking the action that you want to, and self-limiting beliefs can prevent you from excelling in your life.

If you want to correct any of these negative emotions, then this is the perfect book for you. The first step to fix a problem is to accept that you have a problem. Kudos to you—you understand the different aspects of life that you want to fix. The next step is to understand the primary cause of these issues. Once you understand that, the easy part is to fix them. It is quite easy to fix the way you think.

You need to understand that your brain is like any other muscle in your body. With a little training and conditioning, you can unleash your true potential. Most of us don't work at our maximum potential, and often there are certain things that prevent us from doing so. These reasons can be external as well as internal. It is a general misconception that you cannot control the way you think or feel. On the contrary, there are many things in life that you cannot control, but you can certainly control the way you think and feel. You cannot control the external events in life, but you can control your response to those events. The course of your life often depends on your responses to situations around you.

NLP is a technique that helps you reconfigure the way you think and process things. It is a very simple tool that helps you change the way you deal with your thoughts and emotions. At times, all that you need is a little perspective to change your life, and NLP will help you with that.

In this book, you will learn about the history of NLP; its benefits; its core concepts; ways in which you can use it in your daily life; tips to overcome limiting beliefs; steps to adopt a positive mindset and unleash the power of the subconscious mind; and other topics that will help you lead a successful life. If you want to help yourself to resolve these issues quickly and fulfill your goals easily, then this is the perfect book for you.

So, if you are ready, then let us start without further ado.

Chapter One: What is NLP?

In this chapter, you will learn about the origins and the history of neuro-linguistic programming.

Inception

Frank Pucelik, John Grinder, and Richard Bandler conducted studies on three therapists and this led to the inception of neuro-linguistic programming. They referred to it as a behavioral model at the time.

It all began when Richard Bandler met Frank Pucelik. Frank had returned from the Vietnam War and was quite traumatized by all that he had gone through. He found a friend in Richard Bandler. Bandler was a warehouse assistant at Bob Spitzer's publishing company, Science and Behavioral Books. As their friendship blossomed, Bandler and Pucelik decided to help each other rebuild their lives by copying the approaches mentioned in the transcripts and tapes of Bob Spitzer, most notably those of Fritz Perls (the founder of Gestalt Therapy). Initially, their only aim was to improve their own lives and they did not do it for any theoretical reasons.

The two of them started to practice Gestalt Therapy with a group at the University of California. After a while, they were joined by a young linguistics professor named John Grinder. He approached them with a couple of his observations and questions that marked the beginning of a long and successful relationship between these three that led to the birth of the modern-day topic of neuro-linguistic programming. When they started to work together, they began using their collective skills and creativity to analyze and model the works of other people like Fritz Perls and Virginia Satir, who is also known as the mother of family therapy. They studied the rate of success of these two therapists and wanted to emulate their studies by understanding the reasons for their success. They were introduced later on to Gregory Bateson, who introduced them to the works of Milton Erickson, a psychiatrist who specialized in medical hypnosis and family therapy.

Expansion of the Development Team

Once the ideas and insights started to flow, the core team was interested in trying them on others. This led to the expansion of the team as other friends joined them and helped them develop their work. Some of them were David Gordon, Robert Dilts, Judith DeLozier, and Leslie Cameron. There were many others who joined them subsequently and this highly creative group developed NLP.

Most of the methods that were developed during this phase are still a part of NLP training programs. Some of these techniques are anchoring, calibration, reframing, sensory acuity, and representational systems. A couple of other personal change methods, like the Change Personal History and New Behavioral Generator, are still practiced.

NLP and Tony Robbins

Business guru, Tony Robbins certainly seems to know it all. Tony Robbins achieved all the success that he did in his life with the help of NLP. In fact, NLP transformed his life. Robbins believes that knowledge isn't power, but it is merely a source of potential power.

Whenever you read something inspirational, have a rather brilliant idea or come across some life advice and tend to feel inspired and you vow to change your ways. The reality is quite different, isn't it? The inspiring moment passes you by, you don't do anything to follow through with it and it makes you feel frustrated. Therefore, it is not about what you know, but how you execute it that makes all the difference in life.

We are all usually conditioned to listen in a passive state. For instance, we might sit at the desk looking at the laptop, stretch out on the couch reading a book. Passive learning certainly doesn't inspire any action. Robbins recognized this pattern and decided to change it. He understood that the only way in which he can break this pattern is to use the information and act on it. The one thing that differentiates him from others is that he always follows through.

Robbins had a rough childhood and whatever he achieved in life, it was due to his determination and hard work. Success can mean different things to different people, but there is one equation that everyone can use to achieve the success that they want.

The first step is to understand your purpose.

Once you understand your purpose, you need to adopt the right mindset to stick to your goal. Robbins insists that you need to focus on the things that you want and not what you don't want, since energy follows focus. It is essentially the **law of attraction**.

Once you adopt a **positive mindset**, the next step is to take action. You need to consciously work towards your goal.

If you want to be successful, you need to work towards your goal and you also need to check your progress along the way. Assess your progress and proceed accordingly.

If you can change your approach towards how you deal with life and the problems you face, achieving success does become simpler.

These are the simple steps that Robbins followed which made him successful in life.

Books, Workshops, and More

The first publication on this subject was a two-volume book, *Structure of Magic I and II*. This book is considered to be one of the most difficult books to read about NLP because of its highly theoretical nature. During 1973-1976, when the group's creativity was at its peak, they developed new ideas and techniques, experimented with the concepts they already knew, conducted workshops, and wrote their first books, *The Structure of Magic I and II*. They also published *Patterns of Hypnotic Techniques of Milton H. Erickson, MD, Volume 1* in 1975, focusing on Erickson's use of language, their initial model. Apart from this, they also released *Erickson* Volume 2 in 1977.

John O. Stevens transcribed and edited the tapes from their earlier workshops and published them under the title *Frogs into Princes* in 1979. Just like most books on NLP at that time, the book also focused on therapists who wanted to help their patients. These books challenged the traditional way of thinking and offered practical alternatives. These books successfully convinced several therapists to try NLP. Bandler and Grinder continue to organize workshops about NLP throughout the seventies and, towards the late seventies, they had become so popular that their workshops were always packed.

The Commercialization of NLP

The creativity and excitement about NLP inspired a lot of people during the seventies, but this excitement was quickly overshadowed in the eighties. People started to care more about commercial issues, and there was a lot of debate about who was doing it right and who owned it. During this time, Grinder and Bandler parted ways and there is said to be some bitterness between them. They worked on developing their own ideas of NLP from that point on and soon NLP became a way to gain power over one's life as well as that of others. It was no longer a simple route to self-discovery but was considered to be a product that could be marketed to people who wanted quick results.

The Current State of NLP

At present, there is no one particular type of NLP. After Bandler and Grinder parted ways, different NLP camps emerged. The two obvious camps consisted of supporters of Grinder and Bandler, but that was just the beginning. Soon, there were Tony Robbins camps and Lesley Cameron-Bandler camps and many others followed suit. NLP was coming of age and all this diversity reflected its growth.

NLP is more of a movement than an ideology these days. It refers to a body of ideas and knowledge that are constantly developing and diversifying. It is a wonderful and creative concept and one person cannot claim ownership of it. NLP is a personal concept that everyone individualizes to suit their needs.

Uses of NLP

You can use NLP in your personal and professional life.

Personal Life

Communication helps you express your feelings and is an extremely important aspect of any relationship. You can learn to avoid unnecessary fights or misunderstandings so that you have some peace of mind. Not just that, positive communication will bring you closer together as a family and will help you lead a better life.

NLP will teach you to value yourself. Perception of yourself plays a critical role in how you respond to things. Usually, people tend to be a little hard on themselves.

If you want success, then you need to love and accept yourself. You need to accept your thought process and learn to evaluate it as well. You must not beat yourself up for the negative aspects and must instead work to change them.

NLP will bring about an overall change that is quite positive. It will help create an ideal relationship between you and your family members that is devoid of all unnecessary tensions. The rapport that you share with those you love will help strengthen your self-confidence.

Professional Life

Professionally, you can attain a lot of benefits by implementing NLP. For starters, it is a good technique that you can use for solving problems. One of the most important tasks that you will be faced with in any professional setting is solving problems. In fact, if you can effectively solve problems, it is your chance to shine and get noticed. You might be able to impress your boss and even get a promotion. To do this, you need to know how to use NLP to solve problems effectively. Communication is critical, and you need to communicate effectively with your colleagues and coworkers, listening to their feedback before you can decide on a solution.

With NLP, you will be able to easily manage different people in your office. Personnel management can be cumbersome, but it is an important aspect of your professional life. If you want to be successful at work, then you need to be able to successfully manage people and make sure that everyone is on the same page. NLP will teach you to be patient and lead the way. You will find it rather easy not just listen to everyone, but to make others listen to you as well.

Leadership skills are important, especially if you wish to see yourself progress. NLP will teach you the necessary leadership skills to move ahead in life. You will be able to take the right action at the right time and make others follow it as well. Apart from this, your ability to communicate effectively with others and your team will help you become invincible at work. Once you program your brain to work efficiently and remove all obstacles, then you will be able to achieve your targets rather easily.

Social Life

You can use NLP in your social life as well. NLP helps with networking. Once you know how to read someone else's body language, verbal cues, and nonverbal cues, you can communicate effectively. Effective communication is the easiest way to network with others. NLP will help you make new friends and also hold onto the ones you already have.

NLP will help you increase your social responsibility. As you know, it is important for you to give back to society. You can contribute in any which way you like as long as you think it will help you establish a positive impact. Again, it is not limited to just these benefits. You will learn about the many other uses of NLP.

Chapter Two: Identify & Evaluate

Everyone has negative and positive thoughts throughout the day. The positivity quotient in your life depends on the way you deal with the negative thoughts. You can ignore such thoughts, accept them as truth, or confront them. These negative thoughts can weigh you down and suck the life out of you.

In this section, you will learn about the different reasons for all the negative thoughts that you think.

Worry About the Future

Everyone is scared of the unknown, and since you cannot predict your future, a common fear is the fear of the future. People have been continually trying to predict future since the beginning of time. They have tried different things like looking at cracked turtle shells, observing the way birds fly, and the different constellations and positions of stars in the sky. People tend to be scared of the future and all that it might bring.

Will your future bring you fortune or misery? With the advancement of science, people can successfully predict certain short-term outcomes within a closed system like the weather or the elections; however, the average person spends a lot of his or her time worrying about what might or might not happen in the near or distant future.

A lot of people try to maintain a positive outlook about the future and think that they will succeed or achieve the goals that they have set for themselves if they keep trying and don't give up. Well, that's one set of the population that manages to keep a positive outlook, but the rest worry about the future, and the fear of failure is quite real. We all tend to waste a lot of our time and energy thinking about scenarios that might or might not happen. A simple analogy will help put things in perspective for you. The way we worry about the future is similar to paying interest on a credit card that you have yet to use.

You need to understand that the future doesn't exist yet. The fear of the future stems from the fact that we don't have any control over it. One of the easiest ways in which you can regain some control in your life is to plan for the future. You can create a step-by-step plan for yourself. No plan can help you predict the future, but a plan of action can help you regain some control over your life. You can make short-term as well as long-term plans for yourself. A plan will help reduce the fear of future and it will, in turn, reduce any negative thoughts that you have about the future.

Worry About the Present

It isn't just the future that we worry about; we worry about the present too. We worry about the things that are happening or aren't happening in our lives. Worry is a mere extension of fear, and this fear can have a crippling effect on your life. For instance, you might worry about what your kids are doing at school, your finances, or even your work. You may worry about something as simple as whether you locked the car door or not. Phew, that's a lot of worries that we carry.

Imagine how productive your day would be if you didn't worry so much. Well, the good news is that there is a simple way in which you can combat all this fear that you experience. All that you need to do is create a daily schedule for yourself. When you have a schedule to follow, then you can increase your productivity and concentrate on all those things that are important.

Shame in Your Past

We all tend to do things that we aren't proud of. In fact, we might do various things that we find embarrassing. We all make mistakes, and some of those mistakes can haunt us in our present. Well, you cannot let your past control your life. You need to understand that your past is a part of your life and you cannot do anything to change your past. All that you can do is learn from your mistakes and prevent them from happening again. Think of your past as a valuable lesson and nothing else. Your past does not define you. All that you do in your present will shape your future, but your past has no role to play in your present. Instead of worrying about every mistake you have ever made, think about the ways in which you can fix them and learn from them. It is time to regain control of your life and live in the present. If you live in the past or the future, and all that you do is worry about them, you will end up with a list of self-limiting beliefs that will prevent you from attaining any form of success in your life.

You need to understand that your thoughts shape your life. You can control your life and, in fact, you are the only one that can control your thoughts. If you think positive thoughts, you will feel good about yourself, those around you, and life in general; however, negative thoughts can make you feel bad and can disrupt your productivity. Imagine how productive your life would be if you didn't spend your time worrying about negative thoughts.

The easiest way to deal with negative thoughts is to understand their root cause and replace them with positive messages. For instance, if you feel stuck, or if you face an impossibly difficult obstacle, then instead of thinking that you must give up because you cannot deal with it, you can replace this negative thought with a positive one like "maybe I need to change the way I am looking at the problem and try a different approach."

Your thoughts have the power to control and change your life. Therefore, it is important that you make sure that you are in control of them and not the other way around. You cannot get anything done in life if you allow negativity to hold you back.

Chapter Three: The Power of the Subconscious Mind

When you are learning how to drive a car, in the initial stages you tend to be really focused and alert. Your mind will be fully involved in the task at hand, which is driving. After a while, when you have mastered the skill, then you will notice that you needn't be 100 percent focused on driving. Instead, you can listen to music or even talk to others while you are driving your car, without losing control of the vehicle. So, what does this mean, and what part of your mind is controlling the activity you perform? Has this activity been delegated to some other part without your conscious knowledge?

If an object comes near your eyes, then even before you are aware of what exactly has happened, you will blink. How did your body generate this reaction? When you accidentally touch a naked electrical wire or anything hot, what's that mysterious force that is responsible for you pulling back your hand immediately, before you have even managed to figure out what's going on? Why is it easier to change some of your behaviors and habits, even though you want to consciously change all of them? Who or what is responsible for this? Who oversees all these actions and reactions?

The mind is made up of two parts—the conscious and the unconscious mind. Understanding the difference between these two forms the crux of trying to understand human behavior. When you are performing a task and are aware of what you are doing, then such an action will be the action performed by your conscious mind.

Human beings tend to have a very limited attention span. The conscious mind is responsible for learning the task that is required to be performed repeatedly, and then it hands over the reins to the subconscious mind so that the conscious mind will be free to learn other tasks or concentrate on things that require immediate attention. For instance, when you are brushing your teeth, your conscious mind can drift away, and you might start remembering the things that you did all day long or think about the things that you haven't done yet. When this happens, your subconscious mind takes over the activity of brushing your teeth. Any activity that is dull, repetitive, and habitual, like brushing your teeth, will be unworthy of your conscious mind and its attention can be instead focused on thinking about more important functions that need to be performed.

The conscious mind functions as a filter and a logical processor of the information that you receive from the external environment. Based on this information that you receive, your beliefs are formed and then stored in your subconscious mind so that your behavior that is consistent with such beliefs is being carried on its own.

If someone asks you what two plus two is then you will use your conscious mind to answer the question. Similarly, when someone tells you that the earth is flat, then this information will be processed by your conscious mind and interpreted by it, only to find the answer that the earth is spherical and therefore your conscious mind will reject that information, filtering it before it turns into a belief.

If you think of your conscious mind as a filter, then your subconscious mind is the recorder. It is subtler, and the psychology of an individual revolves almost entirely around it. You might have some idea regarding situations in which your subconscious mind comes to the forefront. As mentioned earlier, when you touch something hot, before you even realize it, you will pull your hand back within the blink of an eye. It is a reflex action and is governed by the subconscious mind. The conscious mind always requires some time for processing and therefore is comparatively slower. The subconscious mind is fast and automatic in nature.

The subconscious mind can be perceived as a video recorder that absorbs all the information that you have been exposed to so far. It includes all your experiences, skills acquired, and also your evolutionary history! All this information is too much for your conscious mind to hold; given that it must constantly deal with the present moment, it will be necessary to create a storage system for holding onto all the information that you have acquired. Your subconscious mind is this storage unit.

The human brain tends to work on thought patterns that are nothing but programs that have been embedded into the neural network. You might observe that there is a definite pattern to some of the thoughts that have been produced by your brain. For instance, your brain might be currently involved in the habit of creating a negative pattern of thinking and it will lend a negative flavor to all the information that is being interpreted by it. In such a case, your subconscious mind is looking at reality through the lens of negativity and the root of all this negativity will be a subconscious belief present in some so-called "core" negative thoughts.

The main problem with such subconscious patterns is that you tend to take them for what they seem to be and start believing that they're the absolute truth. However, the truth is simply that the subconscious patterns are the thought patterns that have been through your mind so many times that they have attained an automatic mode of functioning. You can rid yourself of all this negativity in your subconscious mind by not paying any attention to them.

All the thoughts that are running on "automatic" mode form your subconscious mind. All these subconscious thoughts can be observed when the awareness of your mind has been deepened and you can observe the way these core thoughts are essential to most of our perceptions and interpretations. The only obstacle is that, because most of these subconscious thoughts are running automatically, you might presume that they are true and make them a part of your identity. You need to remember that all these core thoughts embedded into your subconscious were all "new" thoughts at one point in time. Some of negative subconscious thoughts are "I will always remain fat, irrespective of what I do"; "I cannot trust anyone"; "I am not good looking"; "and I am not smart enough to make money," and so on. You might have similar negative thoughts at one point of time in your life or another and these thoughts are now running on automatic mode. These core negative thoughts color your perception of reality with negativity.

You need to understand that there is no truth to any of this negativity. Negative thinking only helps foster more negativity and it stops you from moving towards well-being in life. You need to let your awareness deepen and start seeing through all the negativity that exists in your subconscious. It is the only way in which you can get rid yourself of all the negative patterns that you have come to believe in.

Your subconscious is responsible for managing the energies of your heart and it takes this job very seriously. The subconscious mind speaks in a language that consists of physiological feelings and emotions that can be transmitted throughout your body.

The primary directive of your subconscious is your survival. When it thinks that you are incapable of handling disappointment, fear, or any other negative emotion, it immediately takes over. The first reason why you must influence your subconscious is that it helps in providing the much-needed assurance that you can handle feeling vulnerable without being overwhelmed by it. If your perceptions tell you that you cannot, then your subconscious automatically shifts into protective mode. Its secondary directive is to make sure that you thrive. You are designed in a way to not merely survive but so that you are driven by an inner force that motivates you to thrive. You are designed in an exquisite manner to serve a twofold purpose of connecting in a way that's meaningful and also of being your true self while you are in the process of relating to others and life alike. The subconscious shapes your behavior. If you want to thrive, you need to know how to calm yourself and to assure yourself when your fear of survival surfaces, like feelings of rejection, abandonment, or even inadequacy. If you don't feel safe enough to love somebody, then your body will automatically go into "automatic" mode to protect itself.

Infinite riches are present all around you; you just have to open your mental eyes to be able to see for yourself the treasure chest of infinity that is hidden within you. Everything that you need to live a glorious life is within you; you just need to tap into this hidden resource. There are different ways in which you can awaken the power of your subconscious mind. You can access your subconscious by visualization, meditation, dreaming, and so on. In the coming chapters, you will learn about the different NLP techniques that you can use to reprogram your subconscious.

Chapter Four: NLP Training

NLP stands for neuro-linguistic programming, and these are the three core concepts that you need to learn about.

Neuro

Neuro stands for anything that is related to the brain. You have probably come across the concept of neurology at some point. Neurology refers to the study of the brain. On any given day, all our senses work together to help us pick up different stimuli from our surroundings. It can be the odors you smell, the sounds you hear, textures you feel, or even the sights you see. All the senses pick up these stimuli and relay them to your brain; your brain then generates an apt response. The human mind consists of two parts—the conscious mind and the subconscious mind. The conscious mind helps you make all decisions and governs your senses. The subconscious mind is more like an autopilot mode where you don't need to instruct your brain. Even if your subconscious mind helps you perform certain tasks automatically, you still need to consult your conscious mind daily.

What if you can reduce some of that load on your conscious mind? What if you can empower your subconscious mind to make a lot of your decisions? It will certainly make your life easy, won't it? NLP helps your conscious mind converge with your subconscious mind.

Your mind will be able to relate and respond faster to things that are similar in nature. It will be like collecting all the information that lies in your brain and sending it to specific folders that will keep the information safe for a long time. You need to simply extrapolate the information and apply it to the different situations that arise in your life.

Linguistic

The next core concept of NLP is linguistics. Linguistics refers to the study of languages. You cannot communicate effectively if your language skills aren't adequate. If others cannot understand what you are saying, or if you don't understand what they are telling you, then how can you progress? Language barriers can be annoying, especially if they are internal in nature. Human beings are amongst the most expressive creatures on earth and it is quite a shame if we are unable to effectively express our thoughts and feelings. If you want to get your point across, then you need to improve the way you speak. You need to put some effort into establishing better communication skills. At the same time, you need to be good at internal communication as well. Internal communication is critical, and you need to be able to express yourself quickly so that you can take immediate action. If your mind tells you one thing and you do something else, then things will never work in your favor. You need to be able to think clearly and express yourself clearly as well.

Programming

The third concept is the programming. Programming refers to the bifurcation of information and the process of sending such information to different folders in your brain. You need to program yourself in a manner that is conducive to productivity and which helps you make the most of your skillset. When we are young, our minds are fresh, impressionable, and can capture a lot of information. Not just that, but we can also remember things for longer. However, with age, this aspect of our mind starts to change, and it starts to become difficult to process and store information. You can fix this problem with NLP. NLP will help you not just acquire information, but also divide and store it in a simple manner in your memory. Once you understand these core concepts, you can learn about the techniques of NLP. You need to understand that your brain is like any other muscle in your body and you can train it. You can train yourself to be goal-oriented and your mind will not rest until you achieve your goals.

Techniques

Association – Music

For a lot of people, music is an important part of their life. The genre of music doesn't matter; it can be anything that you enjoy. Music tends to have a sway over us that not many things do. It can also influence the way a person feels. It is one of the reasons why music therapy is quite popular. Music helps with our feelings. This is the reason why it is a technique of association included in NLP.

This exercise is about linking a particular song with a feeling of confidence and boosting your self-esteem in this manner. Different people tend to have different feelings about a song; you probably have a song that makes you feel like you are on top of the world. Take a couple of minutes and go through your playlist and find a song that makes you feel confident or inspired. Once you choose a song, you simply need to hum it or sing it whenever you feel down. If you want, you can always pretend to play an imaginary guitar to feel better.

The Trigger

This is a visualization exercise. You need to find a quiet and comfortable spot for this exercise. Now, sit down and close your eyes. Make sure that your breathing is regular, and calm your mind. When you feel calm, open your eyes and try to visualize a mirror image of yourself in front of you. The image that you visualize is self-assured, successful, and reacts differently to things. Focus on this image and study how it behaves.

After you have analyzed this image thoroughly, it is time to put yourself in its shoes. Feel its strength coursing through your body and feel just as confident as that image. This is going to be your trigger from now on. Whenever you want to feel powerful again, repeat this exercise again. The more you practice, the stronger it will become.

Daily Affirmations

Start your day with some daily affirmations. It is the best way to make sure you start your day on a positive note and ensure that you don't miss the opportunity to feel confident daily. You need to make some time for yourself in the morning and think about all the good things about yourself. You must remember that you are the only one that has the power to do what you want, and you have the key to make yourself feel good about yourself. If you want to achieve something, then instead of telling yourself that you will get there, you need to feel like you are already there. Feel like you are the person that you want to be and have achieved the things that you want to.

Kill the Voices

We all experience moments of weakness, where a nagging voice inside our heads tells us that we aren't good enough. It keeps reminding us that someone doesn't like us or that we haven't achieved anything yet. This little voice is really good at spouting destructive thoughts that can remove all traces of motivation that we might have.

Now try to think of the last time you heard this nagging voice in your head. Do you recognize this voice? Is it yours or someone else's? When you have a clear idea of whose voice it is, it is time to change the voice.

This exercise is pretty simple and helps kill that nagging voice in your head. Think of different scenarios and put the voice in such scenarios to render it ineffective. Think of how the voice would sound if it belonged to Donald Duck or any other Disney character. Try to imagine a funny scene where the speaker of the voice is trying to sound serious but cannot pull it off. It will help reduce the effect the nagging voice has on you. It is quite like the manner in which the wizards in Harry Potter defeat a Boggart. The Boggart can materialize their worst fear, and when they imagine it in a funny context, the Boggart loses all its power.

The Whiteout

We all have memories that can surface at inappropriate times, make us feel uncomfortable, and prevent us from giving our best.

We have memories that can surface at the most inappropriate times and make us feel uncomfortable, therefore inhibiting us from giving our best. They are deeply rooted in our subconscious because we have had a bad experience associated with them. The whiteout technique aims at enabling you to stop thinking about such memories at will.

First of all, think of a memory that makes you feel uncomfortable. It can be about a time you embarrassed yourself or when you performed exceptionally badly at something. Once you have the image established clearly in your mind, literally turn up the brightness of the image quickly. Do it very fast, so that the image goes absolutely white.

After this, pause for a second and think of something entirely different.. Repeat the process in quick succession at least six or seven times, and then pause to see what happens. When you will think of the uncomfortable memory again, either it will whiteout all by itself, or you won't be able to see it clearly. Adding a sound effect to the whiteout process can help.

Make sure to pause between each cycle so that your brain doesn't create a loop of the image and the whiteout.

Grounding

This is another basic NLP technique which is really important to learn before you work on some other advanced techniques. It helps you get your confidence issues sorted out and develop a solid foundation from which to work upwards. For this technique, you must be barefoot, but if you can't do that, make sure you are not wearing high heels.

Stand up straight and keep your feet shoulder-width apart and completely flat on the ground. Then move your hips forward slightly and feel your stomach muscles going slightly tense. Your shoulders and arms will be a little loose and your thighs will tense up slightly. Now slightly unlock your knees but don't bend them, and take deep, long breaths, keeping your eyes focused ahead of you. Focus your attention on a point a couple of centimeters below the navel and notice how you feel.

Practice this posture a few times every day, and once you are comfortable with it, try moving around in it. Make sure you are breathing correctly as you move around, and maintain the posture. It will start feeling natural in a while and will help you stay mentally and physically grounded in the reality around you.

Take Words at Face Value

One of the secrets of getting really good at NLP is to take what people say quite literally. It can seem really absurd to some people. After all, we don't always exactly mean what we say. Some things are said just for dramatic value, while others are intended to stress something.

But if you really want to understand the psychology of someone you are talking to, you have to take them literally. People will tell you all you need to know in just the first couple of minutes. You just have to exhibit openness and ask the right questions. For example, if someone tells you they just can't envision themselves losing weight, you must not try to convince them that they can. Instead, you can try and make them see things from a different perspective.

See, people don't like to "lose" things. If that is what you set as a goal, you are bound to fail in most cases. People also don't process negatives as well as they process positives. So telling someone not to think about an elephant will result in just the opposite. It is all wired into our neurology.

Experimentation

The way our communication works is deeply set into our subconscious. When we talk, we subconsciously have a goal in mind, whether we are aware of it or not, and all of our communication is aimed at fulfilling that goal, even if we don't consciously frame our responses.

Try to remember your last leisurely telephone conversation. You will notice that you were not paying much attention to the conversation at least half the time. Your mind was still forming coherent thoughts that manifested into proper replies. This is because language, vocabulary, and grammar are deeply embedded in your subconscious mind.

To become good at communication, you have to experiment with this. Think of yourself as a baby who is still learning and has no concept of failure. Try different phrases and words as you interact with someone you trust, maybe a fellow NLP-practicing buddy. Notice how you get better with time.

Anchoring

A really useful NLP technique for inducing a certain mental state or emotion is anchoring. It can help you enter a mental frame of happiness, relaxation, focus, or anything else you desire, at will. This technique usually requires a touch, gesture, or verbal cue to be used as an "anchor." This anchor acts as a bookmark for you to recall an emotion or state of mind at will whenever you want to.

To understand how the process of anchoring works, let's take a look at an example. For this, first of all, you need to think about a time when you felt really happy. Try to remember one such memory. It can be a time when you won a race that meant a lot to you, or when you had a baby, or maybe when you had your first kiss. Anything you consider a really happy moment will do. Now try to think of the moments before that moment. What happened before the happy moment? Try to create a story leading to that particular moment, and picture it in your head, recalling everything you felt at that time. Try to be as vivid as possible.

When you are at the pinnacle of such feelings, take the index finger and middle finger on your left hand, and place them in your right hand. Then give two gentle but quick squeezes to the fingers. When you squeeze them for the second time, try to picture the happy moment in a larger frame, as if it were closer to you than before. Imagine the feeling growing exponentially and getting stronger inside you.

After this, it is only a game of repetition. Try to describe the feeling again, recalling exactly what you felt at that moment. Then squeeze the same two fingers with your right hand again, and make the picture larger during the second squeeze. After a while of doing this, you will notice that the happy feeling doubles all by itself, without you having to force it to grow. Your progress with this technique will become even faster if you can imagine the feeling really clearly and remember the moment very vividly. Repeat this process at least five times and you will start to feel the effects soon.

Now you have laid the anchor. When you have become adept at this technique, it will become extremely easy for you to recall this anchor at any time by squeezing your fingers twice. You will feel happy instantly just by recalling the anchor.

Pacing

Pacing is a technique that you can use to influence others. When you use this technique, you can enter the other person's model of reality on their terms. It is quite similar to walking next to someone at their own pace. Once you have paced them, and have managed to establish a rapport and have displayed that you understand them, the next thing you need to do is lead them. You essentially use the rapport that you have built from pacing to influence someone else.

For instance, if you want to convince someone to act in a particular manner, the first thing that you need to do is understand why they act in the manner that they do. Once you try to understand this, you can then work on establishing a rapport with them. You need to find some common ground and use that to understand the other person. Once the other person realizes that you both think alike, they will automatically become more receptive to your suggestions.

The Pizza-Walk

From early on, we are taught to think of mistakes as dangerous. It is part of our social conditioning. And for this reason, our nervous system protects us from dangerous situations. What we must understand is that making mistakes is an extremely important part of learning. If you want to be skilled at NLP, you have to give yourself the chance to fail.

A problem many people face when they want to do something is hesitation. To remove hesitation, I like to suggest a method called the Pizza-Walk Experience. It costs almost nothing and can be done anywhere. This exercise will help you let go of all the unnecessary hesitation that holds you back from doing your best.

Think about some of the areas in your life in which you hesitate. After this, go to any commercial space of your choice, like a restaurant or a gas station, and ask for something completely absurd which you are sure you won't find there. Keep a straight face when you request it, and be polite and non-threatening. Repeat this process at least twice in the following week. Notice the change in your responses in situations where you might have hesitated in the past.

It is really that simple. Hesitation is one of the greatest barriers to learning, and with this technique you can completely remove unwanted hesitation in any part of your life. You want to ask out a girl you really like but are hesitating? You want to apply for the new job in a local tech company but are not sure if you are good enough? Go for the pizza-walk and then see the change.

Mirroring

Mirroring is a simple technique that essentially implies that you need to copy another person. Like the name suggests, in mirroring, you need to copy another person's gestures, tone of the voice, movements or even certain catchphrases.

All humans are hard-wired to like and feel comfortable around other humans. In fact, this is an evolutionary advantage. The closer we live together, the higher are our chances of survival as a species. So, anything that is not similar to you will make you feel uncomfortable. You will feel comfortable only around those with whom you feel like you share some similarity. Mirroring uses this concept.

In mirroring, you need to essentially convince the other person that you are similar to them. It is a simple technique that you can use to influence others. The next time you are around someone you like or feel comfortable with, you will notice that you have adopted certain similar gestures that are mirror images of each other. You don't do this consciously, but it is your subconscious that guides you. When you try to mirror someone during a conversation, then make sure that you don't abruptly start mirroring their gestures. You need to do this slowly and gradually because you are trying to influence their subconscious mind.

Start to slowly copy their gestures until your gestures look like a mirror image of theirs. If they change a specific gesture, you can slowly change yours too. If you want to make sure that mirroring works for you, once you know that someone is comfortable with you, you need to try a new gesture. If the other person unconsciously copies your gesture, then it works!

The Swish

The Swish is a rather advanced NLP technique. It doesn't make you forget a bad memory or a negative feeling, but it helps point you in a new direction altogether. You know about the anchoring technique and how you can create anchors to recall certain positive feelings; however, at times, our brain can unknowingly also create negative anchors. When your brain creates negative anchors, then it can trigger unwanted feelings at unfortunate times. The Swish technique helps recode and even delete such negative anchors.

In this exercise, think of an unwanted feeling and image or an associated memory that triggers such a feeling. You need to remove that particular image before the bad feeling sets in. This is the trigger, and you need to replace it with a good feeling and trigger. Place this image such that it is superimposed upon the negative one. You only need speed and not accuracy. Then open your eyes and return to reality. Repeat this at least five times and try to make the Swish quicker each time. After a couple of days, test it to see whether the negative image comes back or not. If it does, then you need to replace it with a powerful image or memory that is more potent.

Chapter Five: NLP – Higher Level of Thinking

Using NLP for Yourself

There are different ways in which you can describe NLP, and this is one of the reasons why it is difficult to find a clear definition of NLP. Also, the name seems pretty vague, doesn't it? Richard Bandler, in one of his workshops, recalled an anecdote on how he came up with the name. Apparently, on one fine day when he was driving, he placed a couple of books about neurology, linguistics, and computer programming on the passenger seat. The police stopped him for speeding. As justification, he tried to explain to the policeman that he was speeding because he was late for a conference. The policeman found this reason dubious and asked him what the conference was about. So, Bandler being the quick thinker that he was, looked over at the passenger seat and replied that the conference was about neuro-linguistic programming. Apparently this is how he came up with the name of NLP. Well, this story might or might not be accurate. In this section, you will learn more about an important aspect of NLP, and that is the mindset.

Even though NLP includes various techniques to change the way you think, the most important concept in NLP is about the mindset.

So, how can you define the term mindset? The best way to describe mindset is as NLP presuppositions. Mindset refers to the assumptions or the principles that a person chooses to adopt in daily life. It is a person's way of looking at the world. The mindset is much more powerful than the simple NLP techniques. In this section, you will learn about using NLP on yourself and others. You can use NLP to influence your mindset so that you feel powerful and in control of your life.

The Map isn't the Territory

It means that our perception of reality is merely a perception and not reality. We often tend to jump to the conclusion that what happens around us is true even when it is often only our interpretation of what we think happened. The difficulty crops up because we seem to react to such events as if they are true. There is a presupposition in NLP that, often, people respond to an experience and not to reality. So, this presupposition reminds you that you need to question what you believe and see if you might have unknowingly distorted it. For instance, if you have an argument with your loved one, in the course of the argument certain heated words are bound to be exchanged. After such an argument, do you start to believe the harsh words your loved one said? You might even hold onto those words and start feeling terrible about yourself. The reality is that your loved one probably didn't mean what was said and you have probably taken it out of context. So, your memory of the reality you think happened, and the reality itself, are quite different.

There is No Failure

Will you feel different if every time you don't achieve your goal, you see that as an opportunity to learn and not a failure? The general conditioning in society is such that if a person doesn't achieve a goal, he or she is deemed to be a failure. Will you start beating yourself about it and start to judge yourself harshly for failing? How about you try to replace this negative thinking with something more neutral and positive? What if every time you don't achieve something, you merely think of it as an opportunity to learn and to do better? A little positive communication with yourself can change the way you view yourself and the world around you.

Communication and its Response

The meaning of communication is the response or the reaction you receive. This one might sound quite tricky. Most of the time, we think that we are being quite clear in the way we communicate, and it seems like our intention isn't being understood or that the message isn't coming across as we intended. It is certainly easier to blame the receiver for the miscommunication; however, it will do you some good if you accept some responsibility in all this. Yes, you were probably clear in what you said, and the other person didn't understand you, but does it matter? If the message doesn't get through, it doesn't matter who is at fault! Isn't it simpler to focus on the best means to get the communication going? This is where NLP comes into the picture. NLP suggests that, the more flexible the communication, the higher the rate of success. There is a presupposition in NLP that, in any system, the element that has the most flexibility will exert the most influence. Therefore, if you are a little flexible in the way you communicate, the chances of you being misunderstood are quite low.

You Cannot Fail to Communicate

Regardless of what you do or don't say, or what you do or don't do, you are still communicating. Even when you are silent and don't express your opinion, you are communicating. Verbal communication isn't the only way to communicate, and nonverbal communication is as important as verbal communication. Your body language, expressions, the tone of your voice, and such are important aspects of communication. You will learn about all this in the next chapter.

You need to learn to establish some positive communication with yourself. If you can influence your mind to think positive thoughts, then your perception of yourself and your life will be positive. You need to let go of any negative beliefs you have and replace them with all things positive.

There are five ways in which you can use NLP to transform yourself for the better.

Dissociate Yourself

Emotional stress can consume you. If you leave it unaddressed, then all the negative emotions can prevent you from evolving and succeeding in life. NLP can help neutralize such feelings and will help you view a situation rationally. When you can view something rationally, or when you can rationalize something, the way you react and respond to it will differ. Instead of letting your anger, worries, or stress get the better of you, you need to learn to dissociate yourself from all that negativity.

Reframe

There will always be situations that will make you feel powerless and when you will be overcome by emotions. In such situations, you need to reframe the content so that you can focus on the things that are important and reduce your stress. You need to remember that there are positive and negative aspects of any situation. If you can merely change the way you view something, then you can shift your focus from all the things that don't matter and can instead concentrate on the things that do matter.

Anchor Yourself

If you want to work on positive emotional responses, even in stressful situations, then anchoring will help you. By consciously channeling a positive state of mind, you will be able to alter the way you feel in any given situation.

Build Rapport

Life is all about establishing communication and building relationships. With the help of NLP, you can build rapport with anyone in your personal and professional life. You will learn to connect with a person through their body language and their communication as well as their breathing patterns. Once you learn to pay attention to the other person, you can easily mirror the way they behave, and it will help you build a rapport.

Limiting Beliefs

The only thing that stops a person from being successful is his or her limiting beliefs. You need to learn to identify limiting beliefs that you might have, and you need to correct them. You cannot simply ignore your limiting beliefs because they can have a crippling effect on your psyche. You are the only one that can change the way you think about yourself. The different NLP techniques discussed in the previous chapter will help you change any limiting beliefs you have about yourself.

Use NLP on Others

People want different things out of NLP, but one common theme among the various expectations people have from NLP is the ability to be able to persuade people better. In this section, you will learn about the different techniques of NLP that you can use to persuade or influence others.

The Antipodean Lilt

First things first, let's talk about the antipodean lilt for a bit. You may have heard of it already, as it is a very popular concept. It's not very potent. It can help you deal better with children, but it doesn't work great for persuasion.

If you don't know what it is, let me explain it in brief. It happens when you let your voice rise in pitch at the end of a sentence. For example, if you say, "I'm going back to Sydney" in a way that the last bit rises up and sounds like a question, it makes you seem unsure. On the other hand, if you say the same part with a lower voice, it sounds more confident and commanding. As a result, the listener feels more confident in what you're about to do, too.

This is a very basic technique that probably won't work on a lot of people, but it still helps to know it.

Embedded Commands

So let's talk about embedded commands. This is one of the simpler yet more powerful techniques. In this technique, you make use of an embedded command in your sentence without being impolite. This makes it difficult for the other person to say no.

Let me give you an example. If you go out often to drink with your friends, think back to one of the times when you were sitting together having drinks and one of your friends said, "Let's have another one." Now, this comes off more like a command, and even though it is fairly polite, it is hard to resist.

So you will most probably oblige unless you really don't want to drink anymore. On the other hand, if your friend asks you, "Do you want another drink?" the power instantly shifts to you, and then it is in your control to decide whether you really want one or not.

The waitstaff at high-end restaurants is often well versed with this technique. They know what to say to get you to buy more. So for example, when you order something like steak and fries, they will often ask you, "What would you like as a starter?" And this makes you instantly look at the menu to find a good starter. Even if you decide not to have one, they at least made you think about it, and that's really their goal. Saying something like, "Would you like a starter?" doesn't work half as well because it just doesn't have that persuasive pull.

Restricting the Choice

This is another one of those really simple yet really powerful techniques. It works by restricting the choice of the listener while giving them an illusion of choice and making them think that they're really in control. Just like in the previous technique, I'll give you an example from the hospitality industry.

When you dine in a fine restaurant, the trained waiter will very politely ask you at some point, "What kind of wine would you like to have?", or "Red or white wine?" These questions are meant to give you an illusion of choice, but really all they're doing is limiting your choice of drinks to the types of wine they have.

If the waiter asks you, "Would you like something to drink?" or something to that effect, it might not have be anywhere near as effective. Now, just like in the previous technique, nobody is forced to accept the offer, but the way the question is posed in the former example sure makes it a lot more difficult for the patrons to resist.

Various fast-food joints like McDonald's and Subway use this technique. While you're ordering a burger, they will very politely ask you something like, "Single or double cheese?" This makes you feel that you are being offered a choice, but what they are actually doing is making sure you don't choose the "no cheese" option.

Something similar is often used when dealing with kids when they're being stubborn. In fact, some smarter parents use it from the get-go so they don't have to deal with stubbornness at all. If you are a parent, you must be familiar with it in some way already.

For instance, when your child doesn't want to go to sleep, instead of trying to scold them or asserting control in a traditional way, what works much better is restricting their choice by distracting them with something else. So you say something like, "Would you like to hear a bedtime story when you have your jammies on?"

In this case, having PJs on is asserted as something that is going to happen either way, and the child only has a choice in whether he wants to hear a bedtime story or not.

"I can, but I'd Rather Not"

This is one of those techniques that people often use with their friends and partners. Everyone uses this, and you might have used it at some point in your life when you wanted to manipulate people into doing what you wanted.

Let me explain how it works with an example. Say you and your friends are going out for the night. You all have a few drinks except for one guy. When you leave, you know it won't be safe to drive while you're inebriated, so you say to your sober friend, "Hey, I can drive if you want," slightly stressing the "if you want" part. This change in tone prompts your friend to step up and volunteer to drive.

If this doesn't seem like the kind of thing you would want to do, maybe you can try a variation of it. When you and your partner are leaving for dinner, you can say, "I'm happy to drive to < the name of the place>" and this conveys to your partner that he or she will be the one driving when you guys come back home.

Know When to Use "and" and "but"

You may not actively realize it, but for a three-lettered word, "but" sure is very powerful. It can change opinions in a matter of seconds. So be very careful of the words that follow. If you understand its power, you can always use it to your advantage.

For example, saying something like, "My friend can do this for you in just a day, but she will charge you $100" makes the listener focus on the latter part: the cost of the work. They might think that a hundred dollars is a bit too much for the work, and so might decline your offer. On the other hand, if you reverse the same sentence and say, "My friend will charge you $100 for this job, but she'll finish it in just one day." This will have a much more powerful positive impact on the listener, as he or she will focus on the "just one day" part. The importance of the cost will be diminished and what will shine is your friend's ability to do the job quickly.

So, to get you familiarized with this, here is a great exercise that you can do with a friend. The rules are:

Each person only gets to say one sentence.

Each sentence starts with the word "and."

After several sentences, change the "and" to "but" and notice the difference. I'm pretty sure that they will have very different impacts on both of you.

Find out What People really Want

This is one of the more advanced persuasion techniques NLP has to offer because what you say really depends on the situation every time, but the rewards are also worth the effort. You get to know what people really want deep inside, and so you can reach common ground accordingly.

It's difficult to get people to disclose what they really want, often because they themselves haven't properly thought about it and they need to be poked a little to think in that direction. What this technique does is remove the need for guesswork on your part. All you need to do is handle the situation properly and people will tell you what they want all by themselves. You just need to gently turn the conversation in the right direction and ask them the right questions.

So, for instance, if you're discussing holiday plans with your friends and you ask them where they want to go, they might respond with an uninterested "I don't know," but they probably do. Now, to know where they really want to go, just ask them a simple question: "Well, if we remove the distance and money factors, where would you like to go then? Think about it." This gives them the chance to really tell you where they want to go, and after that, you can start thinking about the factors that do, in fact, matter (like money and distance) and tailor your response to reach common ground. This will help you all go on a trip where you can do what you all enjoy with a little bit of compromise.

Chapter Six: Explaining VAK

We all use our physical senses to experience the world around us. The five primary senses are sight, hearing, touch, smell, and taste. In NLP, these senses are split into three categories: visual, auditory, and kinesthetic. All the things that we see fall under the category of visual senses; auditory includes all the things we hear; and kinesthetic senses refers to the things that we feel, taste, or smell.

If you want to discover the way in which you use your senses, then take a trip down the memory lane. Remember a pleasant situation, such as a holiday. What is the first thing or sensation that such a memory triggers in your mind? Whatever your first thought is, it will fit into one of the three VAK (Visual, Auditory and Kinesthetic) categories.

For instance, if you remember a beach holiday, for some people the first thing they recollect will be the pleasant blue sky (visual); for others it may be the sound of the waves (auditory). And for others it may be the smell of the sea, the taste of ice cream, or the like (kinesthetic). Your first thought about a memory will help you understand your preferred rep system.

The concept of VAK is a handy tool for interpersonal communication. By using visual words, you can attract someone's interest; with auditory words you can catch the attention of the person; and kinesthetic cues will help you build a rapport. In this section, you will learn about verbal and nonverbal cues.

Nonverbal communication is very tricky to understand. What

we put into words is very clear to understand, but our facial expressions, gestures, and eye contact speak the loudest. Understanding nonverbal communication is a powerful tool that can help a person understand others better and build interpersonal and professional relationships. It can also help you to express yourself better and make connections.

Understanding Nonverbal Cues

While having a conversation with someone, you give away a lot by the way you sit, listen, move, look, and react. The other person can tell whether you are really interested in what they are saying or not, or if you are just pretending to care. When your body language is on par with your words, there is an increase in trust and clarity. When your words don't match with your body language it leads to mistrust, misunderstandings, and tension. For better communication, you need to become more conscious and receptive to the nonverbal cues of others as well as yourself.

Nonverbal cues include the following:

Facial Expressions

Facial expressions are all revealing. Your face expresses emotions more than your words ever can. A smile indicates affection or happiness. A frown indicates disapproval or disappointment. You might say you're doing well, or you're not angry or upset with someone, but your facial expressions may say otherwise. Facial expressions for anger, fear, surprise, disgust, disinterest, irritation, and exhilaration are all very strong and unambiguous.

Eye Contact

Eye contact is another nonverbal communication cue which can give away a lot. When you look into someone's eyes while talking it is a sign of genuine interest and understanding. When the other person fails to make eye contact, is blinking too much, or looks away from you it can mean they are distracted, uncomfortable, nervous, or concealing their feelings.

Mouth

Mouth movements are very important while reading body language. Biting the lips, pursed lips, and covering the mouth are a few signals that convey feelings like distrust, anxiety, and stress.

Posture

Postures say a lot about your state of mind. If you are leaning towards someone while talking it means you are interested in the conversation and attentive. An open posture indicates friendliness and willingness. A closed posture like folded hands or crossed legs indicates unfriendliness and hostility. The way you sit also says a lot; if you are sitting straight, that indicates attentiveness and focus. Sitting with the body hunched forward can mean that a person is tired or bored. Having good posture puts across a good image of you.

Touch

Communicating through touch is very effective. A firm handshake, a warm hug, a pat on the back, and a reassuring arm pat all convey various messages. Touch cues are very subtle and simple to understand. In order to understand and send these nonverbal cues, you need to be emotionally aware during a conversation and be sensitive towards the other person. You need to acknowledge the emotions of others and accurately analyze the cues that are being sent to you. It will help you create and build trust and be responsive to the other person by showing you care and understand.

Tone

The tone of your voice, which means the loudness or the pitch, is also considered a nonverbal cue. The tone of one's voice can have a strong impression on what is being said, when someone talks in a powerful voice.

Nonverbal cues reassure you of what is being said. Make a note of all the cues you are receiving and note whether they are consistent with what is being said. Trust your gut; if you think the cues are not matching up to what is being said then you might be right because nonverbal cues say much more than verbal ones. Learn to understand with your eyes and you won't miss these nonverbal cues.

Understanding Context

While having a conversation with someone, make sure that you observe the body language of the person who you are talking to so you can use your words wisely. Body language can inform you about the comfort level of a person, but that is about it. This is where context comes into play. Understanding context means being mindful of the following things:

The Conversation

You must pay close attention to when the body language of the person changes. What was it that made the person uncomfortable? Was it a question you asked or the topic you were speaking about? Maybe something you said made the other person feel uncomfortable.

The Surrounding Area during the Conversation:

Unless you are in a closed room, all conversations are affected by the environment. Look around you to see the reason why your partner or colleague is uncomfortable. Is there some bothersome noise that is affecting the conversation? Maybe there is an argument going on at the neighboring table, too much of a crowd, or someone your partner knows might've walked in. All these things affect someone's body language and you need to understand that not every person reacts the same way.

Recent Experiences:

During a conversation, you have to keep in mind that your colleague or partner might have had some experiences during the day that might have made them uncomfortable and which may have affected their body language in a negative way. For example, an argument with someone, a rough day at work, health issues, financial troubles, and personal problems may reflect on the body language of a person. If they are still thinking about the stressful situations in their lives, they might appear sad, uncomfortable, distracted, and disinterested.

Take time to determine the reason for your partner's discomfort. Suggest moving to another room or changing the topic and see if that makes a difference. If there is no improvement in their body language, then you can politely ask them if anything is wrong. You might think you are the problem, but there might be something else that is bothering the other person. Offer them some food and beverages and talk about something fun and interesting instead of the same mundane topics. Analyzing and understanding context may seem like an impossible task but with practice, you will get better, and it will become your most valuable skill.

The next time you are having a meeting with your boss, colleagues, or even when you're on a date or out with a friend, watch out for these cues to effectively read people.

Smile

Know a fake smile from a real smile. A real smile will light up the person's face and cause crinkles near the eyes. Your eyes cannot lie, so next time you want to know if someone's smile is genuine, be sure to watch the crinkles near the eyes.

Eye Contact

Eye contact is another important aspect when you want to read someone. Eyes are very expressive and are considered a window to the soul. If the person is looking into your eyes and talking, then it means they are comfortable with you. When you are having a conflict with someone and they cannot look you in the eye, it means they are hiding something from you.

Jittery Movements

When someone repeatedly touches their face, hair, and neck, it means they are nervous and are scared of disapproval. Fidgeting with an object while talking also signifies restlessness and distraction. Clenching the jaw, tightening the neck, or furrowing the brows are all signs of stress and anxiety.

When someone copies your body language, it is a sign of agreement and comfort. This is especially a good sign during negotiations as it shows you what the other person is thinking.

Posture

Slouching while sitting, and droopy shoulders, are signs of low self-esteem and confidence. Such people have trouble expressing their feelings. Sitting upright shows confidence and enthusiasm. You cannot feign interest, as your body language will not match your words.

Placement of Legs

When someone is shaking their leg while talking to you, it means that they are nervous or uneasy. This is a common habit especially during interviews and creates an impression on the interviewer. This is a sign of insecurity and shakiness, which is not very well appreciated.

Placement of Hands

The placement of hands also says a lot about a person's state of mind. When a person has his or her hands on the hips while standing, it means they are enthusiastic, interested, and energetic. Hand gestures while talking means that the person is trying to explain and express feelings and ideas.

Be aware of the surroundings and context when you are reading someone, as body language is just going to give you a hint at what the person is thinking and feeling. For in-depth analysis, you have to take into account the context and apply it accurately.

Facial Expressions

A person can convey volumes through their facial expressions. A smile shows approval or happiness. A frown, on the other hand, shows disapproval or indicates that the person is unhappy. At times, facial expressions might reveal what the person is truly feeling. When someone says they are fine, but they have a small frown on their face, their words are certainly contradictory of what they are feeling. A couple of emotions that can be expressed through facial expressions include happiness, sadness, anger, disgust, surprise, fear, confusion, desire, and contempt. The expression present on a person's face can help you in determining whether they mean what they are saying or not. Facial expressions are part of a universal form of body language. It is quite difficult to control facial expressions when a person is feeling extreme emotions. You can gauge what a person is saying by paying close attention to their facial expressions.

Eyes

Eyes are considered to be the windows to the soul. Eyes are capable of revealing a lot about a person's thoughts and feelings. When you engage in a conversation with someone, observe their eye movements. This must be a general part of your communication process. A couple of things that you must look out for are whether the person is maintaining eye contact, is averting his or her gaze, has dilated pupils, and is blinking either normally or rapidly.

Gazing

When a person maintains eye contact while conversing, it shows interest and implies that the person is paying attention;

however, prolonged eye contact can be perceived to be threatening and intimidating. Breaking eye contact frequently or looking away indicates that the person is distracted, is uncomfortable, or is trying to hide something.

Blinking

Blinking is quite natural; however, blinking too much or too little can signify different things. If a person seems to be distressed or uncomfortable, the person will blink a lot and quite rapidly. Blinking signifies that the person is trying to control what they are truly feeling. For instance, a poker player might blink deliberately and less frequently to hide his or her excitement about the hand he or she has been dealt.

Size of the Pupil

The dilation of the pupil is a very subtle nonverbal gesture. The level of light in the surroundings often causes the pupil to dilate. Even different emotions lead to the dilation of people. When a person is attracted to someone else, their pupils dilate. This shows attraction and arousal and gives rise to the popular phrase "bedroom eyes."

Mouth

The movements of the mouth can also help in reading a person's body language. For instance, chewing the bottom lip indicates insecurity, fear, or worry. Covering one's mouth might be an effort made to politely cover a yawn or a cough; however, it can also be an attempt to stifle disapproval or judgment. One of the greatest signals while interpreting what a person is saying is a smile. A smile can mean various things depending on whether it is genuine or not. Pay attention to the following signals while analyzing body language.

Pursed Lips

While conversing, if someone purses their lips, it shows disapproval, distaste, or even distrust.

Biting of the Lip

Shows anxiety, worry, or stress.

Covering of the Mouth

This is often done for hiding an emotional reaction, like trying to hide a smirk!

A slight change in the mouth is a subtle indicator of what the person is truly feeling. If the corners of the mouth are turned upwards, the person might be feeling optimistic or happy, and if they are turned down, it shows disapproval or sadness.

Gestures

These are perhaps the most obvious signals used. Waving of arms, pointing towards something, or using the fingers for indicating numbers are amongst the most commonly used and easy to interpret gestures. Here are a few gestures that can help you in getting a better understanding of what a person is saying. A clenched fist shows that a person is angry. The thumbs up and thumbs down gestures signify approval and disapproval respectively. The "v" sign made by just lifting the index and middle fingers to form the letter "v" signifies victory or peace.

Arms and Legs

The crossing of arms shows defensiveness, and the crossing of legs indicates discomfort or dislike. When a person has a smile pasted on their face but is standing with their arms crossed, their body language certainly doesn't back up that smile. There are certain subtle gestures that are made by the widening of arms to assume a commanding position or for minimizing the attention of others. When someone is standing with their arms placed on their hips, it shows that a person is ready, in control, or it can also suggest aggressiveness. Tapping of fingers or fidgeting with them shows impatience, boredom, and restlessness. The crossing of legs shows the desire for privacy, and clasping of hands behind the back indicates anger, anxiousness, or utter boredom.

Postures

The way a person holds his or her body is an important part for analyzing body language. Posture refers to the overall physical form of the individual and the manner in which they carry themselves. A lot can be inferred about a person's characteristics from their posture like whether the person is confident, open, dominating, or submissive. When someone sits with his or her back upright, it shows that the person is paying attention and is focused on what is going on. Hunching or slouching while sitting implies that the individual is bored or indifferent towards what's going on.

Open Posture

This involves keeping one's torso open and exposed. This shows that the person is open, willing, friendly, and approachable.

Closed Posture

If a person is hiding his or her torso by hunching forwards and keeping the hands and legs crossed, it can be an indicator of hostility, unfriendliness, or even anxiety.

Personal Space

What does personal space mean? Did you ever feel uncomfortable when someone gets a little too close to you? Personal space refers to the social distance that an individual like to maintain with others. The physical space between two individuals can provide a lot of information if you know what you are looking for.

Intimate Distance

If the physical distance is between six to 18 inches, it shows that the individuals share a close or an intimate relationship. This happens while whispering, hugging, or touching.

Personal Distance

This is the physical distance that is usually maintained while talking to family members or close friends and it ranges between 1.5 to four feet. The closer a person stands to another while communicating, the closer the bond that they share.

Social Distance

Social distance is the distance that is maintained with acquaintances. When an individual knows the other person fairly well, the distance maintained is between four to 12 feet. Depending on whether or not a person is well acquainted with the other, the distance between them will increase or decrease.

Also, the distance that is maintained can depend on culture. For instance, people from Latin America are comfortable standing closer together while interacting with others, whereas those from North America appreciate more personal distance.

If you are trying to understand the true meaning of what a person is saying, then make sure that you are paying close attention to their body language. A person's body language can give away what they are truly thinking, feeling, or implying; however, while trying to notice someone's body language you need to be observant, but this doesn't mean that you should stare or ogle.

Chapter Seven: NLP and Anchoring

NLP anchors are an easy and quick way to tune into a resourceful state of mind on demand. There is nothing better than feeling positive emotions by simply flipping a switch. In this section, you will learn about the concept of anchoring and the ways in which you can create anchors.

One of the most important tools of neuro-linguistic programming that you can use to increase your self-confidence, interest, and make yourself feel relaxed is anchoring. It is a simple technique that assists you to alter any negative or unwanted feeling into something that is positive and resourceful in no time. Whenever you create an NLP anchor, you establish an involuntary response to stimulus so that you can immediately feel the way you want, whenever you want. In NLP, the word anchoring refers to a process that enables you to associate an internal reaction with an external trigger or an internal trigger so that you can easily and quickly reassess your reaction or response to such a stimulus.

Anchoring is a technique that might seem quite similar to the conditioning technique that Pavlov developed; at least they seem similar on the surface. In the conditioning technique that Pavlov used, he managed to create an association between salivation in a dog on hearing a bell ring. Pavlov associated the ringing of the bell to feeding his dogs, so the dogs automatically created an association that the ringing of bell signified their feeding time. Eventually, Pavlov noticed that merely by his ringing the bell, his dogs started to salivate, even when he didn't feed them. The theory rests on the premise that an external stimulus or cue can elicit a behavioral response. The association formed is said to be spontaneous and not based on choice. The behaviorist's stimulus-response conditioning formula helps condition a subject's response or behavior to a specific stimulus.

In NLP, anchoring is a form of relative conditioning that includes links between various other emotions and experiences instead of restricting it to external cues or behavioral responses. For instance, the reaction or internal feeling you experience whenever you remember a particular picture will become an anchor for you. The tone of your voice can become an anchor that associates the tone to a specific feeling like excitement or confidence. With anchoring, you have the option to establish, as well as re-trigger, an association for yourself. Instead of your reaction being an unconscious response, anchoring is a tool that helps with self-actualization. Anchoring is an effective tool that helps you create and restart a mental process that is associated with learning, creativity, and the ability to concentrate, as well as other important experiences.

The comparison of an anchor used in NLP has certain significance attached to it. An anchor helps to stabilize a boat or a ship so that it doesn't float away and stays rooted to a spot. An anchor is dropped by the crew of a ship or a boat to keep it stable and hold it in a specific spot. In NLP, an anchor is a psychological anchor that helps generate a response and isn't a mechanical stimulus. If we extend the previous analogy of a ship, then in terms of human psychology, the anchor refers to an experience in our consciousness. Anchors are points of reference that help find a specific experience and hold our concentration there and prevent it from wandering away. Visualize what it will be like, in an instant, if you go from feeling apprehensive to feeling confident and capable while in a stressful meeting when all eyes are focused on you or when you are dealing with a problem. That will certainly simplify your life, will it not?

The concept of an NLP anchor is quite simple. It refers to a connection that exists between a stimulus and an emotional response of an individual. NLP anchors work because when a person starts to relive an intense emotion, and at the peak of that experience uses a particular stimulus, then the individual forms a neurological link between the two events. As mentioned earlier, it works exactly in the manner in which Pavlov conditioned his dogs to salivate upon the ringing of a bell. We all use NLP anchors most of the time and we do it unintentionally. For instance, a big shiny yellow M can be an anchor for a cheap and crappy meal or it can signify a tasty, feel-good meal. When you are driving, and you approach a set of lights that suddenly turn red, it can be an anchor for either road rage or a sense of mild frustration, according to your temperament at that instant.

The good news about anchors is that you have the option of anchoring specific triggers to an emotionally positive state. It means that you can feel confident, happy, and energetic, or experience any positive emotion whenever you want to. To enable this reaction, you need to be able to use your imagination and have around ten minutes to spare. According to the strength of the memory that you use as an anchor, an anchor can last you anywhere between a couple of weeks up to a month at a time.

It is quite wonderful if you are in control of your state of mind. Being control of your state of mind gives you the power to change it whenever you want. Imagine that you can feel happy, confident, relaxed, or experience any other positive emotion at will. Imagine you can change the way you feel at will. If you want to do this, then anchoring is the best technique. The way we react can be intentional as well as unintentional. For instance, if you touch something hot, do you quickly pull your hand away or do you contemplate the action that you need to take? You obviously pull your hand away instantly. This is an unintentional response that is a part of your subconscious mind. Similarly, when something is anchored, then your reaction to such a situation will be automatic and you won't have to contemplate what you need to do. Such an association can be both good as well as bad. For instance, some food that your grandmother cooks can remind you of your childhood. Or maybe, every time you pass by a place or see an object, it might remind you of a bad experience.

The thing about anchors is that they can be both positive as well as negative. Like mentioned earlier, we create certain triggers unknowingly. These triggers can be both positive as well as negative. It is important to get rid of any negative triggers and replace them with positive triggers. For instance, if you pass by a certain place or wear a certain t-shirt, does it remind you of a bad phase in your life? Perhaps you were out of a bad relationship and that place or that item of clothing reminds you of those bad times? If you are slouching on the couch for long, does it make you feel lazy and slightly depressed, and then you start to binge on junk food? Well, do you ever experience the urge to binge on unhealthy snacks when you feel low? This is an example of a negative anchor that your mind created. You can create positive anchors and in the same manner, you can break free of negative ones. **Positive psychology** is the basis of anchoring and you will learn about establishing positive anchors in the coming section.

Anchoring is a simple technique that will allow you to create or break certain associations consciously. It uses different stimuli like sound, image, touch, smell, or even taste to deliberately trigger a response that is consistent. In fact, knowingly or unknowingly, we use this technique in our daily lives. For instance, brands use anchors while advertising. They use anchors that associate their products with a, particularly positive feeling by using pictures of happy people, enjoyment, or even success. The downside to this technique is that it can create negative associations. For instance, if you wear something during a particularly painful event, then you will start to feel uncomfortable every time you wear that item of clothing. If you wear a particular shirt while undergoing dental surgery then, whenever you wear that shirt afterwards, you will be reminded of the discomfort you experienced. Your mind has managed to form an association between that item of clothing and an unpleasant event. Most of the anchors are created accidentally; however, you can deliberately create positive anchors to remind yourself of something good.

You can create an anchor in all perceptional systems. You can create visual, auditory, kinesthetic, olfactory, and even gustatory anchors. A visual anchor uses images that can bring back memories or feelings associated with a color that can make you experience a particular mood. An auditory anchor can be a song that might remind you of a specific event—like whenever you hear a siren, you tend to feel alert. Kinesthetic anchors like a hug or the feel of cold breeze can remind you of someone special or a specific place. Olfactory anchors trigger your sense of smell. For instance, the smell of a specific perfume can remind you of someone. Gustatory anchors trigger your sense of taste. For instance, the taste of a specific dish can remind you of your childhood and such.

Anchoring is used to access feelings, a state of mind, or resources whenever you want so that you can replace an unwanted feeling with something more pleasant. It can also help you control your emotions and reactions. When you can control your emotions and reactions, you can have better control over the situations in your life. For instance, if you are stressed or anxious, then you can use a happiness anchor to access a happy memory that can instantly make you feel better about yourself.

Now that you know what an NLP anchor is, the next thing that you need to know is how to create anchors for yourself. There is a simple acronym that you can use to remember the parameters to create an anchor. The acronym is I-TURN, which stands for:

- Intensity

- Timing

- Uniqueness

- Replicability

- Number of times.

Now, let us understand these parameters to create a powerful anchor. The first parameter that a memory needs to meet, if you want to use it as an anchor, is intensity. If you want the anchor to be powerful, then the memory that you use needs to be powerful. All that you need to do is opt for a strong memory and slightly tweak the submodalities (a subset of the modalities— visual, auditory, olfactory, gustatory, and kinesthetic) of the memory to make it intense.

The second parameter that you need to concentrate on is timing. The idea is to use an anchor when the happy feelings associated with the memory are at their peak. If you do this, then you will be able to generate a strong response. The best way in which you can perfect the timing of the memory before you use it as an anchor is to relive the memory in your mind. Go through the memory and note the moment when your emotions are at their peak.

The third parameter that a memory needs to meet if you want to use it as an anchor is its uniqueness. The uniqueness in this context refers to the stimulus and the meaning that you want a specific trigger to have. For instance, a popular trigger is rubbing the earlobe or rubbing the fingers together. You can select any trigger that you want, but make sure that whatever the trigger is, you can do it in public without offending anyone.

The fourth parameter is replicability. Replicability means that you must be able to replicate the anchor in the same manner that you created it and it must not be a problem. If you plan to use the anchor in public, or you know that you might need to use the anchor in a public setting, you need to make sure that it doesn't include any inappropriate movements. For instance, the trigger cannot be something like touching yourself inappropriately.

The final parameter is how many times you use it. The higher the number of anchors you stack, the better. As with everything else in your life, the more work you put in, the better your performance will be. It is ideal to spend about 30 minutes setting an NLP anchor. If you do this, then the anchor you create will be quite powerful. If the thought of spending 30 minutes on this task doesn't appeal to you, then keep in mind that once you create an anchor, you don't have to redo it again. So think of the time that you spend on this task as an investment. However, if you really don't have any time to spare, then you can spend about ten minutes and create an anchor, but then you will need to spend ten minutes every week refreshing the anchor.

Steps to Create an Anchor

Now that you know what an anchor is, and the parameters that you need to keep in mind while setting up an anchor, the next step is to create an anchor. It is quite easy to create an anchor. Follow the simple steps discussed in this section to create one.

Pick a Memory

The first step is to pick a memory. Don't just pick a random memory. The memory that you opt for must have strong feelings associated with it. If you want an anchor for confidence, then you need to select a memory of something that made you feel confident. If you want an anchor for motivation, then select a memory that you find motivational. If you cannot pick a memory, or if you feel that you have never felt like this, then you can create an anchor by imagining yourself in a resourceful state; however, an anchor is most powerful if the instance or the memory that you use is something that you have experienced.

Association

Relive the memory by seeing it through your eyes. The more vivid and specific your imagination, the better the anchor will be. Close your eyes and reimagine the situation or experience that you want to use as an anchor. Try to experience your emotions as vividly as you can.

The Feeling

Once you start to experience a positive feeling, create a trigger. A simple trigger is to rub your fingers together. So, whenever you rub your fingers together, you trigger a specific memory. The feeling that you want to re-experience needs to be positive.

Release

When the emotion you experience is at its peak, release the trigger. It can take some practice, but you will understand what to do after a couple of tries.

Test

To break the state, you need to do something completely unrelated for about thirty seconds. After this, you need to test your anchor. So, if your trigger is to rub your fingers together, then when you rub your fingers together you need to experience the same feelings that you did in your memory.

Repeat

To make it work, you need to work on the anchor. You need to repeat it at least thrice to make the anchor stick. Initially, it might take you a couple of tries to trigger a memory. With a little practice, you can see the results almost immediately. Work on creating a strong association between memory and the trigger.

Chapter Eight: NLP for Procrastination and Negative Beliefs Specifically

NLP for Procrastination

Here is a simple NLP exercise that you can use to overcome procrastination.

Close your eyes and picture yourself working on a task and the actions that you need to take. Picture all the steps that you need to accomplish to complete the task. Now, see your expression in your mind's eye. Do you look happy and relaxed? How does this make you feel?

Now, imagine the same instance, but this time you need to see it through the eyes of your future self. What will you see, hear, and feel in this instance? Imagine how your future self will feel when you have accomplished the task.

You need to now make this image slightly larger or move closer. Adjust the brightness if you want to intensify the feelings you experience. If you feel that the emotions are fading away, go back to the previous configuration. This is quite similar to editing a picture. Focus, adjust, crop things, or do anything to make the visualization seem more real.

Once you do this, think about the three specific benefits that you have gained by completing the task at hand. You might or might not have reached the goal, but you have completed the task. Maybe this process was a learning experience for you; you might have discovered some strength of yours that you weren't aware of, or you might have discovered that you like something.

Consider these three benefits that you will obtain if you overcome procrastination and work on your goal.

Now, consider the three benefits that you will not obtain if you let procrastination get a hold of you and you don't do something.

Once you do all this, it will give you the perspective that is necessary to work on the task and overcome procrastination.

NLP to Overcome Negative Beliefs

You can start developing your mental strength by setting reasonable goals for yourself. It is not just about setting goals, but about taking the necessary steps to achieve your goals as well. If you want to start working towards your goals, you need to start applying yourself. It means that you will have to ask yourself, even when you are bored or going through some turmoil, to stick to the plan until you have accomplished the goals you have set for yourself. It will not be an easy feat, so don't let it scare you. Practice makes perfect, and this age-old adage is true! Keep practicing, and you will get better! If you have set some big goals for yourself and they seem impossible, try breaking them down into manageable steps that are doable. For instance, if you want to become assertive, then your first step must be to learn to speak up for yourself at least thrice every week. These instances can be major or minor, but you have to speak up for yourself. Develop a "stick with it" mindset. Even if you face an obstacle or a setback, keep trying and don't give up. Start being resilient and don't worry about the troubles you come across. The goal is to keep going until you have achieved what you want. Think of all the failures as an opportunity to learn—and please do learn from them. Every day is a new day, so don't let the troubles from your past sneak up on you.

Negativity can sneak up on you quite quickly. It can stem from a negative emotion that you are harboring within yourself, or it can be because of something external such as negative feedback or toxic people around you. While certain things are beyond your control, the one thing that you can control is the way you feel about yourself and your life. Don't let any negativity live within you. You cannot control what others think about you, but you can certainly control the way you feel about yourself. There are different ways in which you can manage all the negativity. You can start by identifying and challenging such negative thoughts. You can reduce your interaction with harmful and toxic people. If you think you are in a toxic relationship, learn to break free of it. Don't entertain negativity in any form.

Make use of positive self-talk for building up your mental strength. Making use of positive affirmations will help you in developing a positive outlook while getting rid of all negativity around you. Take a couple of minutes and look at yourself in the mirror and say something positive and motivating to yourself. You can say something that you believe in, or something that you would like to be true.

When you learn to control your emotions instead of letting them control you, you are giving yourself an opportunity to weigh your options before deciding on a particular choice. Take a minute and count to ten before you let a negative emotion boil over. It might sound like a cliché, but it does work. Before having an emotional reaction toward something, take a moment to gather your thoughts and react accordingly. You can try practicing meditation as well, and it can help you in maintaining your calm. Meditation can help you in staying objective while providing you with the necessary time for making sense of your thoughts and emotions. Instead of reacting immediately, you can weigh your thoughts and emotions and then think of your next step.

If you are always sensitive to the petty annoyances and verbal barbs or taunts that we all tend to come across daily, then you will end up becoming quite bitter. Also, you will be wasting a lot of your precious time and energy thinking about unnecessary things, which don't matter at the end of the day. When you start spending time thinking about all such things and start paying attention to them, you are making them a significant problem that will increase your stress. Learning to adjust your attitude can help you in letting these petty and trivial issues go without increasing your level of stress. You are not only preventing the wastage of your valuable time and energy, but you are also saving yourself the trouble of having to deal with extra stress. Instead of stressing yourself out about all these things, you must develop a healthy routine of thinking about the things that are bothering you, then take a deep breath, calm down, and once you are calm, think of the best way in which you can deal with that issue.

For instance, if your spouse keeps forgetting to put the cap on the tube of toothpaste after using it, understand that such a thing isn't as important to your partner as it is to you. If this bothers you, think about all the other things that your partner does for you that make you feel good and in comparison, you can certainly let this small flaw of theirs go. Don't try to be a perfectionist, at least not all the time. When you do this, you are setting high expectations for yourself, and these tend to be entirely unrealistic. Try to be realistic while thinking about things and don't let the idea of perfection create any additional stress or burden.

You can make use of a straightforward visualization exercise that will help you in letting go of little things that seem to be bothering you. Take a small stone or pebble and hold it in your hand. Transfer all the negative thoughts that are bothering you into that pebble. And once you are ready, swing as hard as you can and toss the pebble away or into a pond. Visualize that all the petty problems are drowning along with the pebble that's sinking. You are casting away all your negative emotions.

We tend to get so caught up in the problems that we tend not to look at things from a different perspective. A fresh attitude towards existing troubles can help in solving your problems. If you feel like you have hit a dead end with something, take a break and relax. Once you feel refreshed, start thinking of ways in which you can tackle that problem. If you change the way in which you are approaching a problem, you might find a solution to it in no time. Here are a couple of different things that you can try for gaining a new perspective on things.

Start reading. Reading the daily news or a book can help you in stepping into someone else's world, and this serves as a good reminder to let you know that the world is a vast place and that your problems are nothing significant when you think about the entirety of the universe we live in.

All those who are mentally as well as emotionally strong tend to be happy with what they have. They usually have a positive outlook towards life and don't complain much. It doesn't mean that they don't have any problems. Of course, they have problems just like everyone else, but the difference between them and everyone else is that they can see the bigger picture and know that the challenges they are facing are a part of life. Maintaining a positive outlook towards life will provide you with the mental and the emotional strength that you need for tackling any problem you come across. Remember that bad times will pass, and good times are just around the corner. Don't lose hope.

The ability to face reality is a sign of mental and emotional strength. If you are going to overcome a hurdle or a challenge, then you must be able to tackle it head-on. Lying to yourself about your troubles won't make them go away, and you will just end up hurting yourself in the process. If you overeat when you are stressed or sad, accept the fact that there is a problem that needs to be addressed. Don't look for a means of escape, and try being honest with yourself.

Dealing with Life

Whenever you feel that you are stuck in a difficult situation, take a while to think things through. Don't react instantly, and don't be in a hurry to make a decision. It will provide you with sufficient time for your emotions to diffuse and you can start weighing your options with an open mind. It is essential that you do this, regardless of the situation you are in. If you can afford to, then take some time and list the pros and cons of a situation. Make a note of how you are feeling as well. Try finding some positive points about the situation you are in, and this can help in changing your perspective towards things.

At times, the smallest change in perception can make a huge difference. Follow the ten-second rule. Give yourself ten seconds for something to sink in before expressing yourself. Even if your partner tells you that he or she wants to end the relationship, take ten seconds to compose yourself and then respond.

Once you have managed to compose yourself, before you decide on a course of action, think clearly about the circumstance you are in. What happened, and what are the possible options available to you? There will always be more than one path that you can opt for. For instance, let us assume that your friend asks you to do something morally wrong and you are torn between your loyalty to your friend and your sense of morality. So now you will need to weigh the different pros and cons and decide accordingly.

Make use of your inner voice or your conscience for guiding you. Trust your instincts, and you are likely to be correct. At times, the answer might be quite clear and distinct, but it might be hard to do the right thing. Do not let the problem fester into a more significant hassle than it already is. You need to make a call and stick to it. You can always ask others for an opinion and weigh their opinions before deciding; however, remember that it needs to be your own decision and no one else's. If you feel like you are stuck, think about what someone you admire would do in such a situation. The decision that you make must be something that you can live with. Don't do something because someone else thinks that it is a good idea. Do it because you want to.

More often than not, we tend to find that our minds are flooded with a lot of negative thoughts. These negative feelings can become quite powerful when you keep thinking about them endlessly. The problem starts when you start focusing on these thoughts, and they naturally become more powerful. Doing this makes it quite difficult to break free of the mental rut you might be in. In this chapter, you will learn about a couple of simple things that you can do to control your thoughts.

Making a Conscious Decision

The problem is that, at times, we get attached to specific ideas and complications, and we subconsciously derive some weird form of pleasure from going through those issues. If you keep subconsciously inviting such negative thoughts, you will never be able to stop thinking about them. Therefore, the first step is to make a conscious decision to clear your mind and stop it from replaying all the negative thoughts on a constant loop. Be aware of the impact these negative thoughts have on you and prevent them from getting stuck in your mind. Make a conscious effort to stop all the negative thoughts from dwelling in your mind.

Separate Your Thoughts

When you try to stop individual point of views, you will notice that it seems incredibly difficult. This happens because ideas are a significant part of your mental process. The second stage is to separate yourself from your thoughts. Whenever a thought pops into your head, view it as if it was from an external source. It will help in reducing the impact negative thoughts have on your mind. Once you realize that you can, in fact, make this distinction, you can start modulating the ideas you think about. You must be able to control your thoughts, not the other way around.

Who is Thinking those Thoughts?

You need to understand where your thoughts originate. Whenever an idea comes to you, first try to understand the reason why you are thinking that specific view. Realize that your thoughts can be controlled. Whenever a negative thought comes into your head, try diverting your attention towards something positive. If you find that you aren't able to do this, then try thinking about the cause of such a thought.

Chapter Nine: NLP for Fear and Phobias

Overcome Fear and Hesitation

You can use NLP techniques in every aspect of your life. Everyone experiences self-doubt, fears, and other phobias at some point in their life. Even the best of us are bound to wonder from time to time whether we are good enough. You might even worry about whether something you do will make you seem stupid or foolish in front of others. These fears can prevent you from auditioning for a play, prevent you from learning to dance, stop you from speaking in public, or even prevent you from doing something that you want to. Fear is a major obstacle that everyone faces in life. Fear can be real as well as imaginary. Regardless of what it is, fear has a paralyzing effect that can prevent you from achieving greatness in life.

Inaction can breed fear, and the only way to overcome fear is to take action. Instead of taking action or seeking a means to overcome fear, a lot of people hesitate. This hesitation can make all the difference in your life. People usually think "maybe I am not feeling up to it in this instance, or I am not feeling my best and I will do something about it when I feel 100 percent." However, these are just words and that day might never come. A common excuse is a lack of time or the fear of disappointing someone else. There are so many people who want to change their job but are scared of doing so. They often tell themselves, as well as those around them, that they are probably too old to change their job and that it will cost them job security. As you will learn in this chapter, you are never too old to make a change and all the fears that hold you back are nothing more than illusions.

Even if it sounds hard to believe, there seems to be some sort of comfort in not taking any action. Some simply believe that others are successful because either luck seems to favor them or they have some innate ability that makes them successful. If you think like this, then you have a free membership to the club of whiners and envious people. Instead of worrying about the success that others receive and blaming your lack of it on your luck or fate, it is time for you to take action.

If you want to achieve something in life, you need to change and take some risks. There is no reward without risk, and change is essential to growth. If you really want to change the way you think, and you want to let go of all fears that hold you back, then NLP is your answer. There are different positive techniques that NLP suggests that you can use to control your fears and overcome any phobias.

Now that you know what NLP anchors are about, using that technique will come in handy. Once you've practice anchoring, then you can move onto the exercise that's discussed in this section. You can do this exercise on your own, or you can always find someone else to do it with.

The first thing that you need to do is make some time for yourself from your daily schedule and think about an instance where you faced a barrier to something that you wanted to do. Perhaps you couldn't muster the courage to ask for the promotion that you thought you warranted, or you couldn't read the book that was lying on your shelf which you'd intended to read for so long.

Picture that particular event in your mind as clearly as you possibly can. Feel all the feelings and emotions that you experienced. Listen to any sounds that are associated with it. As soon as the image is clear in your head, anchor that feeling to some part of your body.

Think of all the times you had a barrier, and perform the same routine of visualizing it. Experience it, and then stack the anchors in the same manner.

Now, try to think about the frustration or regret you experienced at not doing those things that you wanted to and then stack these anchors as well.

Once you do this, visualize a time when you took the necessary steps and went for something that you did want. You might need to dig a little deep. The specific moment that you are looking for might or might not seem significant. Regardless of what you think about it, it refers to a time in your life when you did something that you wanted to in spite of your apprehensions.

Now, create a large picture of this event in your mind. Experience what you saw, hear what you heard, and feel all that you did. Transform this picture into a movie and see yourself chasing whatever it was that you wanted.

Let this feeling of satisfaction wash over you and as it does, anchor this feeling to a different part of your body.

The next step is to get rid of the first anchor and as you do this, think about all the times when you stopped yourself from going for it. As this feeling bubbles up within you, fire the second anchor and hold these together for a moment and release the first anchor. Now, as you fire the first anchor, hold onto it until it triggers a sense of frustration within you and then fires those anchors. As the feelings continue to build, hold and then release the second anchor. Keep repeating this process until the need to take some action overwhelms you and motivates you to take action.

This is a simple exercise that you can use to overcome any fears you have. There is another exercise that you can try to dissolve your fear and hesitation.

This exercise that you are about to learn was designed by Stephen Ruden and Ronal Ruden. This exercise is known as "havening" and is quite effective.

As with any other exercise, you must first read all the instructions carefully before you decide to start the exercise. If you must, then please do go over it a couple of times to understand it fully.

The first thing that you need to do is think about a barrier that you have and think about how terrible it makes you feel. Once you decide on a specific barrier, then rate it on a scale of one to 10—with 10 being the worst. You need to rate this barrier so that you can measure your progress later on.

After this, clear your mind of all thoughts and start thinking about something that is pleasant. Now, with both your hands, tap simultaneously on your collarbones. Keep your head still, continue to tap on the collarbones, look ahead, and keep your eyes open. As you tap and keep your head straight, look towards your left and then towards your right.

Continue to tap on both your collarbones and keep your head still. Now, move your eyes in a full circle—first move your eyes clockwise and then counterclockwise.

The next step is to cross your arms. Once you cross your arms, lift them up slowly so that each hand of yours is resting on top of your shoulders. As soon as your hands rest on your shoulders, close your eyes.

Start to slowly stroke your hands downwards on the sides of your arms—start at your shoulders, make your way towards your elbows, and then back again. Continue to repeat this motion.

As you continue to stroke the sides of your arms, visualize yourself walking down a flight of stairs. As you walk down the stairs, count from one to 20 with every step that you take. As you reach 20, you can either hum or sing the first three lines of the "Happy Birthday" song.

Now, let go of your arms and let them rest by your sides. Relax your body, slowly open your eyes, and look up. Look up and then down; after, this move your eyes from the left to the right and then back again. Repeat these movements thrice.

Close your eyes and take deep breaths. Inhale slowly and exhale slowly. As you exhale, gently stroke your arms and repeat this process five times.

You can now open your eyes. Think about the barrier you face and rate it on a scale of one to 10. When you are calm and composed, you will notice that the specific block you worried about doesn't seem that scary now. It might not have lessened as much as you want it to, but it still has lessened. You need to repeat this exercise a couple of times, and every time you will notice that the barrier seems less and less worrisome.

You can perform this simple exercise whenever you want to, in any stressful situation. The aim of this exercise is to calm your mind so that you can logically work on overcoming any fear that you experience. As you let the moment of panic pass you by, you can contemplate a rational course of action.

Overcome Phobias

If you have a particular fear or a phobia, then here are a couple of ways in which you can deal with it.

Avoid

Well, the most straightforward way in which you can deal with a phobia is to avoid the thing that scares you. It certainly won't be a problem if you are scared of a great white shark, dinosaurs, or something like that. It will be problematic if you are scared of needles, spiders, or even cheese. You don't necessarily have to be phobic about a tangible thing; you can have a phobia of things that you cannot see but can experience like a relationship or commitment. So, how do you deal with such things? How do you avoid feelings and things related to them? Avoidance is a way to treat the symptom, but it doesn't treat the cause. Avoidance can also at times intensify your fear and that's not something desirable. People tend to go to great lengths to avoid things and this can cause severe disruption in one's life. If you go to great lengths to avoid someone just because you are scared of commitment, you will disrupt your life and will not deal with the issue at hand.

Desensitization

You can desensitize yourself to something that scares you. For instance, let us assume that you have a severe phobia of snakes. Now, you go see a therapist to help you deal with this problem. During the first session, your therapist wanders off to the other side of the room, opens a book, and shows you a picture of a snake from about 25 feet. Your heart might skip a beat or two, but you will be fine. During the second session, the therapist places the book a little closer to you, say perhaps ten feet, and shows you the image of a snake for 10 seconds. After a while, the therapist places the book next to you and you are still fine. After this, the therapist waves a plastic or a rubber snake at you. After a while you get used to it and it will not scare you as much as it used to. You get the idea of this technique, don't you?

The premise of this exercise is to slowly expose you to the thing that scares you and reduce your sensitivity to it. You can use this logic to deal with any problem that you might have in life. For instance, if you are scared of commitments while in a relationship, then the first step is to tell your partner that you love them. Now, give yourself a couple of weeks to get used to the idea before you take the next step. Over the course of a couple of months, you can tell your partner you love them without shutting down.

Flooding

If you think that desensitization isn't doing the trick for you, then the next exercise that you can follow is flooding. Let us continue the previous example of phobia of snakes. The next time you go for a therapy session, imagine that your therapist pulls a lever and you walk into a trap. The trap plummets to the ground and you are fine. You are fine, and you are in a cage. You think everything is fine, and then you look around and notice that you are surrounded by snakes. Placing yourself in close quarters with something you are scared of might overwhelm your senses initially, but after a while, you get used to it.

Another simple technique that you can try is to rationalize your fear. To rationalize something that you are scared of, you need to examine the cause of such a fear. What is it that scares you? Is it the thing, or did you have an upsetting encounter with such a thing? If you can address the issue that gave birth to your phobia, you can successfully tackle your phobia. If you are scared of commitments, take a moment and think about the reasons why commitment scares you. When was the first time you realized that you are scared of commitments? Is there something in your past that caused this fear? Perhaps it was a failed relationship, or perhaps you experienced a rather harrowing childhood. If you can identify the reason for your fear, you can rationalize it and tackle it. Examine your life; examine the fear and the cause of such fear. When you do this, you can easily overcome your fears.

Chapter Ten: Other Ways to Support Positive Thinking

Get Sufficient Sleep

Getting sufficient sleep will not only keep you healthy but will make you happier as well. The age-old saying "Early to bed, early to rise, makes a man healthy, wealthy, and wise" is true. Make sure that you go to sleep early and get about seven to eight hours of undisturbed sleep. If you cannot wake up on your own in the morning, then you can set an alarm. Give yourself an hour to unwind before going to bed. You can read a book, watch some TV, go for a walk, or do anything that will relax you. It isn't just about the number of hours you sleep, but the quality of sleep that matters as well.

Healthy Eating Habits

Avoid all sorts of processed foods that are full of sugars, unhealthy fats, and undesirable carbs. Instead, opt for healthy foods that are rich in fiber, nutrients, and essential macros. Healthy food will nourish your body and will leave you feeling energetic. Unhealthy foods like chocolate or chips can be replaced with some fruits or nuts. Here are a couple of simple tips that you can keep in mind to make sure that you are eating wholesome food.

Have complex carbohydrates like whole grains and leafy vegetables instead of starchy foods like bread, pasta, or pizza. Your meal must be rich in protein because it not only leaves you feeling fuller for longer, but is good for you as well. Stay away from all processed foods and instead opt for healthy treats like kale chips, nuts, fruits, or anything that isn't full of saturated fats and trans fats. Replace sugary drinks with water (sparkling or still). Create a food plan for yourself. If you are interested in cooking, then learn to experiment with recipes and cook something different. Healthy food doesn't have to mean bland salads, so keep an open mind and try your hand at cooking. If you plan your meals in advance, then you can do all the meal prep on your day off; this simplifies the entire cooking process.

Drink Plenty of Water

Water is good for your body and drinking plenty of water will make your skin clearer and will flush out all the toxins from your body. Make it a habit to have at least eight glasses of water daily. If you want to, you can add some flavorings or electrolytes to your water to spruce it up. Slices of lemon, different berries, a handful of mint leaves, or slices of cucumber can be added to water to make detox water. By following these five simple tips, you can trick yourself into drinking water.

Drinking water needs to be convenient. Carry a water bottle or a sipper with you wherever you go. If a water bottle is handy, it is more likely that you will drink water. Instead of sugary sodas and sweetened beverages, you can have unsweetened water-based drinks. Instead of a Frappuccino, have a cup of Americano. Make it a point to drink a glass of water before and after your meals. Set a goal and measure the amount of water you are drinking daily. If you keep a track of your water intake, you will be motivated to drink more. Don't forget to drink water even when you go out drinking with your friends. Don't let your body get dehydrated.

Don't Forget to Treat Yourself

This doesn't mean that you must spend your next paycheck on a pair of fancy shoes or a handbag. Instead, you need to do things that will nourish your soul. There might be a book that you have been meaning to read but haven't gotten around to. So, take a day off and do that. If you like gardening, then try growing your own kitchen garden. Take some time off from this busy world, put away all the gadgets, and instead do something that you enjoy.

If you are feeling stuck with your work all the time, then take a break. Take a couple of days off and go somewhere. You don't have to plan an elaborate or a fancy vacation. You can go hiking or even fish for the weekend. Do something that you have been meaning to do but haven't found the time for yet. Book a day at a spa for yourself or get a massage. Pamper yourself once in a while and connect with your inner self.

Friends Matter

Spend some time with your friends. Your true friends are the ones that have been there for you regardless of the ups and downs in your life. True friends are like a life jacket; they will keep you afloat. Don't get so busy in your life that you don't have the time for your friends. Tell them how much they mean to you and show them that you love them. Always stay in touch with your friends.

Keeping in touch with your friends is one of the easiest things that you can do to enrich your life. You can stay in touch with them by using different social media applications. Make it a point to call your friends once a week and talk to them. It isn't just about messaging them. Make plans to meet them once a week and at least twice or thrice a month. When you are out with your friends, put your devices away. Focus on the conversation and spending time with them instead of checking your phone constantly.

Smile Often

Don't let small issues bog you down or make you feel blue. Not everything in life is to be taken seriously. Try looking at the positive side of any situation. You always have a choice; you can either feel hurt or you can let it go. Don't be pessimistic and learn to smile. A smile is contagious, and it helps improve your overall mood.

Make it a point to smile as soon as you wake up. This will provide you with a positive mindset while starting the day. Remind yourself that you must smile often in a day. Set reminders or think about the things that make you smile. Create certain cues to smile. Make it a point to smile at everyone you make eye contact with. Smile often and the same will be reciprocated. Think happy thoughts and you will automatically start smiling. Try doing this and you will see a positive change.

Enjoy Your Hobbies

A hobby is an activity that makes you happy and acts as a stress-buster. You might like to paint, draw, dance, sing, play a musical instrument, collect things, or do something else. Spend some time doing things that make you happy. If you don't have a specific hobby as of now, then it isn't too late to cultivate one.

Stay Away from Negative People

You don't need any form of negativity in your life. Stay away from all those who are trying to bring you down. Surround yourself with positive people and those who mean well. The company you keep matters a lot. You will be happier if you are around happy people. Surround yourself with people who are successful, ambitious, and positive in general. Don't argue with a pessimist. It just makes things worse. Instead, let it all go. A negative person feeds off negativity and by indulging in an argument, you are just adding onto it. Just stay silent and let the negativity pass you by.

Dealing with negative people might be quite difficult; however, don't let them get to you. If you can find it within you to give them some love, then do it. If you can't, then stay away from them. Be the bigger person and show them love. You never know the reason for their negativity. If someone you know seems to be upset, perhaps you can offer them a hug or get them a glass of water. If you aren't able to do any of the above-mentioned things, then it will be best if you just stay away from such people. Maintain your distance, and be civil to them if need be, but that's about it.

Don't Forget the Important Things in Life

Regardless of how successful you are or how tough your life is at present, don't forget those who are important. Success won't mean a thing if you cannot share it with someone you care for. Popularity, fame, and wealth don't matter. These things are transient, so don't forget those who are permanent in your life like your friends and/or family members. Spend more time with your loved ones. You can arrange a weekly gathering and meet your friends or your family members. Develop a tradition of a weekend brunch or barbecue that will allow you to spend time with those you love. Even watching a movie with your loved ones will make you feel happy.

Chapter Eleven: Maintaining Positivity

Overcome Obstacles

Focus on the Result

If you are putting something off, then one way in which you can change your thinking is by focusing on the result. Think about how you will feel once the work is done well. Visualization is a great tool and will help reduce the anxiety that you might be feeling before getting started. A positive mentality makes it easier to get things done.

Define What You Want to Accomplish

For instance, if you have a goal that you want to write your autobiography, then make sure that you are setting a deadline for it as well. A deadline can be a tremendous motivating factor. Precisely define the goal that you want to achieve. It is highly unlikely that you will stay motivated when the goal is vague.

Make a Note of the Reasons

There might be different reasons for doing something. If you don't have a reason for doing something, it is meaningless. Having a reason will provide you with the necessary motivation. Understanding your reason will make the task meaningful.

If You Don't Do It

It might or might not work for you. At times, the fear of not doing something and the disappointment that will follow can be motivating. Think about the worst possible outcome if you don't do a particular thing. You can make use of those feelings to propel you forward.

Setting Mini Goals

You can always break down your goals into smaller goals. Doing this will help in making your goal seem more achievable. Not just that, but it will help you in measuring your progress as well. Setting and accomplishing small goals will provide you with the necessary motivation to keep going.

Scheduling

Regardless of what your project is about, you must schedule some time for it. Write it in your calendar, set a reminder, and treat it like any other regular appointment. You will not be able to achieve all your goals if you don't commit to the project. If you feel that you are having some trouble sticking to the schedule, then think about all the reasons for which you are doing it.

Marking Your Progress

Create a checklist of all the mini-goals you have established for yourself. This will help in keeping track of your progress. If you feel that you are lagging somewhere, you can put in some extra effort to improve your performance and progress.

Staying Consistent

If you want to be consistent, then here are a couple of tips that you can follow.

Make a to-Do List

Making a to-do list is very helpful. Take a sheet of paper and write down all the things that you have to complete in a specific. You can either do this as soon as you wake up in the morning or on the previous night. So, when you wake up in the morning, you will have a sense of direction, and you will know what needs to be accomplished by the end of the day.

Create a Reward System

Always create a reward system for yourself. Regardless of whether you have completed a small or a big task, you must still reward yourself for completing your work. The reward system doesn't have to be an elaborate one.

Breaking Up Your Workday

Breaks are essential, and you will need a couple of breaks while you are working. It is quite difficult to work efficiently for prolonged periods of time without any breaks. A small break will make you feel refreshed, and it will improve your ability to concentrate as well.

Don't Indulge in Any Activities that will Waste Your Time

Avoid, or at least try reducing the time you spend indulging in any addictive time-wasting activities. It can be anything. Even something as simple as playing a game on your phone can be quite addictive, or constantly checking your social media feed. These activities will not help you accomplish anything, and they just eat into your working hours. Set certain limits. You can do these things while on a break, but not while you are working. Get your work done and then you have plenty of time for all the other activities.

Tackle the Tough Tasks First

There will always be a couple of tasks that you think are tough. It is a good idea to get these tasks out of the way as soon as you possibly can. Don't keep these tasks on hold. Once you are done with these tasks, the rest will be relatively more straightforward.

Discuss Your Goals with Someone

When you tell someone about your goals, you will unknowingly increase your accountability. It is likely that you will finish a task if you have already told someone about it. You get to decide whom you want to discuss it with. Accountability towards someone else will make you want to complete the task at hand.

Kill Procrastination

Figure Out the Reason

When you feel like you aren't in the mood to do something, this is procrastination telling you to take a break. The task at hand can be something very simple or incredibly complex. The reasons for putting off a task can be quite varied. Instead of getting frustrated with yourself and blaming procrastination, you must take a moment and evaluate the situation. Give yourself some time for figuring out the reason why you are procrastinating. This is the first step if you want to overcome procrastination and it is crucial.

Procrastinators tend to concentrate on the short-term gains instead of the long-term ones. Instead, you need to focus on the benefits of completing the task on hand. For instance, if you have put off cleaning out your closet, then imagine how good you will feel when the closet is free of all clutter! Concentrate on this feeling and it will be easier to get things done.

Getting Rid of the Obstacle

Before you get started with a task, give yourself a few minutes and consider the likely obstacles that you might have to face. Then, you can start devising a plan for avoiding or overcoming these obstacles. For instance, you have received an email giving certain instructions regarding the manner in which you are supposed to go about doing a particular task. You will keep going back to read the same email frequently while starting out with that task. This will lead to unnecessary distractions. Instead, you need to print these instructions beforehand. By simply planning ahead, you will be able to avoid procrastination.

Just Get Started

At times, it might seem really difficult to get started with something. Taking the first step might be quite tough, regardless of the task at hand. Just take that first step, and it gets better. When you stop focusing on all the negative things about a certain thing, you can prevent yourself from getting discouraged. When you just dive right in, you will notice a positive change in your mood and this is quite helpful.

Break it Down

If something intimidates you, it is very likely that you will end up putting it on hold for as long as you can. If you can reduce this intimidation, it will be easier to work on something. The sheer size of a project can be an intimidating factor. So, try and break it down into smaller parts. When you do this, the intimidation quotient will decrease. It is easier to tackle smaller tasks.

The Right Environment

Working in the wrong environment will make way for procrastination to creep in. You certainly won't be able to get any work done if you are working in a really loud place, you have your friends around, or you are constantly on your phone checking the latest social media updates. You certainly will not be able to get any work. Your surroundings must help you work and not distract you.

Rejoice in the Small Victories

Always enjoy your victories, regardless of how small or big they are. A sense of accomplishment will help you in keep going. This will help in developing a positive attitude towards your work and will provide you with the necessary motivation to keep going. Striking off simple things from your to-do list can be quite satisfactory.

Be Realistic

When you are setting goals for yourself, make sure that the goals you are setting are realistic and attainable. You will be setting yourself up for failure if you set unrealistic goals. This will increase your negative feelings and you will ultimately succumb to procrastination.

Self-Talk

The more you tell yourself that you aren't supposed to think about something, the more time you will spend thinking about it. This is just how the human psyche works. It becomes almost impossible to not think about it! The trick is to not let this happen. When you feel yourself leaning towards putting something off for a while, you must try and avoid it. Simply shift your attention to something else. For instance, instead of thinking that you aren't supposed to procrastinate, try thinking about how good you will feel once you have completed the task. In this manner, you will be able to take the necessary action instead of worrying about a certain behavior.

Don't Try to be a Perfectionist

Perfectionism is quite a difficult mentality to function with. This all or nothing sort of thinking can lead to procrastination. A perfectionist will believe in only two outcomes. Either something can be perfect, or it will be considered to be a failure. People with this tendency will wait until everything is absolutely perfect to proceed. If it isn't perfect, then it cannot be completed. This mentality can hold you back from not just starting a task, but from completing it as well. Instead of chasing perfection, focus on being better. Strive for excellence, but at the same time, your focus needs to be on completing the task.

Chapter Twelve: Homework

Try these exercises for a week and you will notice a positive change in your behavior.

One Problem per Day

Every morning, select one problem that you want to work on during your spare time. Identify the different elements it is made up of for figuring out a logical solution to it. To put it simply, go through the following questions in a systematic order: What is the real problem? How does this problem obstruct your goals, purposes, and needs in general?

Here are the steps that will help you with problem solving.

Whenever it is possible, try tackling problems one by one. State the problem as precisely and as clearly as you possibly can. Then study the problem to understand its nature. For instance, you will need to figure out the kind of problems that you can solve. Differentiate between those problems that you have control over and those that you don't. Learn to set aside those problems that you have no control over. Think of the information that you will need and actively start looking for the same. Analyze and interpret the information you gather and draw reasonable conclusions from it. Think of the different options you have, both long-term and short-term solutions. Once you know the options that are available, the next step is to evaluate all the pros and cons each of these options offer. Select an approach and follow it. Once you have implemented your plan of action, you must monitor the implications of the same. Depending on how the plan functions, make changes as need be.

Internalizing Intellectual Standards

Universal intellectual standards include clarity, precision, accuracy, relevance, depth, breadth, logic, and significance. Every week, select any one of these standards and try to increase your awareness of the same. For instance, you can focus on clarity for a week, then shift towards precision, and so on. If you are focusing on clarity, observe the way you communicate with others and see for yourself if you are being clear or not. Also notice when others aren't being clear in what they are saying. Whenever you are reading, see if you are clear about the content you have been reading. While expressing yourself orally, or while writing your thoughts down, check whether there is some clarity in what you are trying to convey.

There are four simple things that you can make use of for checking whether you have some clarity or not. Explicitly state what you are trying to say, elaborate on it, give examples for facilitating better understanding, and make use of analogies as well. So, state, then elaborate, illustrate, and lastly, exemplify yourself.

Maintain an Intellectual Journal

Start maintaining an intellectual journal wherein you record certain information on a weekly basis. Here is the basic format that you must follow. The first step is to list down the situation that was emotionally significant to you. It must be something that you care about, focused on one situation. After this, record your response to that situation. Try being as specific and accurate as you can. Once you have done this, then analyze the situation and your reaction and analyze what you have written. The final step is to assess what you have been through. Assess the implications—what have you learned about yourself? And if given a chance, what would you do differently in that situation?

Reshaping Your Character

Select an intellectual trait like perseverance, empathy, independence, courage, humility, and so on. Once you have selected a trait, try to focus on it for an entire month and cultivate it in yourself. If the trait you have opted for is humility, then start noticing whenever you admit that you are wrong. Notice if you refuse to admit this, even if the evidence points out that you are absolutely wrong. Notice when you start becoming defensive when someone tries to point out your mistake or makes any corrections to your work. Observe when your arrogance is preventing you from learning something new. Whenever you notice yourself indulging in any form of negative behavior or thinking, squash such thoughts. Start reshaping your character and start developing desirable behavioral traits while giving up on the negative ones. You are your worst enemy and can prevent your growth unknowingly. So learn to let go of all things negative.

Dealing with Your Egocentrism

Human beings are inherently egocentric. While thinking about something, we tend to subconsciously favor ourselves before anyone else. Yes, we are biased towards ourselves. In fact, you can notice your egocentric behavior on a daily basis by thinking about the following questions:

What are the circumstances under I favor myself? Do I become irritable or cranky over small things? Do I do or say something that is "irrational" in order to get my way? Do I impose my opinion on others? Do I speak my mind about something I feel strongly about? Once you have identified the egocentric traits, you can start actively working on rationalizing yourself. Whenever you feel like you are being egocentric, imagine what a rational person would say or do in a similar situation and the way in which that compares to what you are doing.

Redefining the Way in which You See Things

The world that we live in is social as well as private and every situation is "defined." The manner in which a situation is defined not only determines how you feel, but the way you act, and its implications; however, every situation can be defined in multiple ways. This means that you have the power to make yourself happy and your life more fulfilling. This means that all those situations to which you attach a negative meaning can be transformed into something positive if you want. This strategy is about finding something positive in everything that you have considered to be negative. Try to see the silver lining in every aspect of your life. It is all about perspectives and perceptions. If you think that something is positive, then you will feel good about it, and if you think its negative, then you obviously will harbor negative feelings towards it.

Get in Touch with Your Emotions

Whenever you start feeling some sort of negative emotion, ask yourself the following:

What line of thinking has led to this emotion? For instance, if you are angry, then ask yourself, what were you thinking about that caused the anger you are feeling? What are the other ways in which you can view this situation?

Every situation seems different depending on your perspective. A negative perspective makes everything seem dull and bleak; on the other hand, a positive outlook does brighten things up. Whenever you feel a negative emotion creeping up, try to see some humor in it or rationalize it. Concentrate on the thought process that produced the negative emotion and you will be able to find a solution to your problem.

Analyzing the Influence of a Group on Your Life

Closely observe the way your behavior is influenced by the group you are in. For instance, any group will have certain unwritten rules of conduct that all the members follow. There will be some form of conformity that will be enforced. Assess how much this influences you and the manner in which it influences you. Reflect on whether you are bowing too much to the pressure that is being exerted and whether you are doing something just because others expect it of you.

One Door Shuts and the Other Opens

Take into consideration any negative moment in your life that has led you towards a positive outcome; an outcome that you weren't expecting. Make a note of these things every day.

The Gift of Time

Time is precious. Spending time with someone is the best gift you can possibly give them. So this week, offer the gift of time to three different people. It can be in the form of helping them around the house, taking a person who's feeling lonely out for a meal, or even catching up with an old friend. These things must be done in addition to your other planned activities.

Counting Kindness

Keep a journal where you can write down the kind deeds you performed in a day. Make a note in your journal before going to bed at night.

The Funny Things

Each day, write about the three funny things that you have experienced all day long. Also make a note of the cause of such a funny incident. Was it something you said, observed, or was it something spontaneous?

Letter of Gratitude

Think of someone who has had a positive impact on your life and write a letter of gratitude to that person. If it is possible, you can also deliver it to them in person.

The Good Things

Write about the three good things that you got to experience in a day. Also state the reasons why such things occurred.

Making Use of Your Signature Strengths

Take a VIA survey. This survey will help you in finding your character strengths. Select your biggest strength and make use of it in a new manner. This is a daily task.

If you aren't keen on writing things down, then consider discussing things with someone who is close to you. Talk to yourself about all the positive aspects of your life. Also make sure that you have practiced the above-mentioned steps for at least one full week.

Conclusion

I thank you once again for choosing this book and hope you had a good time reading it. Neuro-linguistic programming is a technique that aims at improving a person's life. It helps a person turn a favorable situation into an unfavorable one. The best part of NLP is that there is no failure. No mistake you make can ever be wrong; it's just a stepping-stone to your improvement. Every mistake you make acts as feedback that you can utilize to further improve your life. This makes NLP one of the best ways to improve various aspects of yourself.

Every person has the potential to succeed in life. All we need is a little push to make us unlock this potential. This is where NLP comes into the picture. NLP is not a tough concept to understand. If you understand what the individual words stand for, then you will know how to implement it in your life successfully. You need not spend countless hours trying to perfect it. Just taking it up and practicing it daily will help you adopt it successfully.

If you want to lead a happy life that's filled with positivity, then you need to adopt a **positive mindset.** Follow the simple tips mentioned here to make sure that you can maintain positivity forever.

You need to understand that you determine your reality. You are the only one that has the power to decide whether your experience is positive or negative. You need to remember that you are the only one that creates **limiting beliefs** for yourself.

You attract what you believe in. **Positive psychology** is about maintaining a positive outlook in life so that you can attract positivity. If you want to attract happiness, you need to think positive thoughts, if you want to achieve success, then you need to think about that success and not the obstacles you might have to face. Use the **law of attraction** to attract positivity into your life.

You need to create a positive morning ritual for yourself. Make it a point to spend the precious morning hours doing something productive and don't waste that time.

More often than not, things don't necessarily go as planned. You might feel frustrated when your plans change or when they don't work in your favor. However, resistance doesn't change anything, and things just go downhill from there. When you start accepting what has happened, only then can you let go of all the unnecessary suffering. You must begin practicing acceptance, understand and adjust yourself to a circumstance, without any conflicting emotions clouding your judgment.

You must live in the present, because that's where everything happens, and it is the only place where you can experience happiness. Your past might be full of beautiful memories, but you cannot get anything from those memories. By living in the past or the future, you forget about the moment that you have in hand. Your present is critical, and you must start living in it as well. Gadgets happen to be a significant part of our lives these days, and social media is an even more substantial part. Your online presence needs to go hand in hand with your offline life as well. Learn to live in the present, physically. It isn't about living in the virtual world all the time; it doesn't make any sense.

Listening and hearing are two different concepts altogether, even though these words are used interchangeably. Listening is a conscious process where you need to pay attention. It helps in establishing a strong bond between people and assists you to live in the present. Therefore, it is an excellent source of happiness. You need to make a conscious effort to be more present while having a conversation with anyone.

Money can help you in buying things, and worldly things will assist in making you feel momentarily satisfied. Why don't you try saving up to 6 months without shopping unnecessarily? You will be able to save a small fortune, and you can make use of that money to travel instead. Instead of filling your life with all sorts of expensive branded products, you must try creating beautiful memories that will make you feel happy whenever you think about them.

Most of us tend to stop making friends as we start growing older. You must always be interested in meeting new people. It will help you in improving as a person, widen your horizons, and ensure that you have a lively social life. Try striking up a conversation with a stranger, and you never know, maybe you will end up with a new friend.

Dreams provide you with the motivation to keep going. Therefore, always try to dream big. Your dream will assist you in finding the one thing you are passionate about. Let yourself dream and have sufficient faith in your ability to turn that dream into reality. You must always spend 5 minutes daily and step into your dream world. Start visualizing about the things that you want to do and how amazing you would feel once you achieve your dreams. Try making your visualization as real as possible, and it will increase your desire to work towards that goal.

Does your present look anything like the future that you have been dreaming about? If not, spend some time and energy thinking about the various things that you can do for ensuring your growth? You don't have to do everything at once. Start by taking small steps, and you will ultimately reach your goal.

If you want to lead a successful and happy life, then you need to make a conscious effort towards it. It takes some time, hard work and effort to change the way you think, but the results will certainly make it worth your while.

The steps and strategies mentioned in this book are all tried and tested and will surely help you get started with NLP. They will also help you stay with the practice.

I wish you luck with your NLP endeavors and hope they bring you success.

Lastly, if you found this book helpful please leave a positive review on Amazon as it is greatly appreciated and keeps me being able to deliver high quality books.

Resources

https://whyamilazy.com/use-nlp-techniques-fight-procrastination/

https://www.the-secret-of-mindpower-and-nlp.com/NLP-techniques-for-dissolving-fear-mental-blocks-and-hesitation.html

https://www.adaringadventure.com/banishing-phobias-and-fears/

http://www.fulfillmentdaily.com/10-habits-to-grow-a-positive-attitude/

https://www.forbes.com/sites/forbescoachescouncil/2018/03/22/10-ways-to-beat-procrastination-and-get-things-done/#346663292902

https://medium.com/the-mission/these-6-powerful-ways-will-help-you-overcome-obstacles-and-reclaim-your-power-b1fabdb8e074

https://www.personal-development-planet.com/nlp-anchors.html

https://www.nlpcoaching.com/7-nlp-ways-train-brain-positive-ways/

https://www.notsalmon.com/2011/07/07/how-to-use-nlp/

https://www.subconsciousmindpowertechniques.com/remove-negative-thoughts-from-mind/

https://www.gaia.com/article/3-ways-to-positively-influence-your-subconscious-mind

https://www.powerofpositivity.com/3-reasons-negative-thoughts/

www.ingramcontent.com/pod-product-compliance
Lightning Source LLC
Chambersburg PA
CBHW072147020426
42334CB00018B/1917